RAINFOREST REMEDIES

D1018961

RAINFOREST REMEDIES

ONE HUNDRED HEALING
HERBS OF BELIZE

Rosita Arvigo and Michael Balick

Text Illustrations
Laura Evans

LOTUS PRESS
Twin Lakes, WI

CHABOT COLLEGE LIBRARY

RS
164
A78
1993

PUBLISHER'S DISCLAIMER
This book is a report on research being conducted by two ethnobotanists
working in Belize. It does not purport to be, nor is it intended to be, any
kind of a recommendation or self-treatment guide for the use of herbs or
indigenous plants. The statements in this book are based on traditional
lore and have been reported in an attempt to preserve and codify
traditional cultural values and information. Nothing should be construed
to represent an attempt to diagnose, prescribe or administer in any
manner to any physical ailments or conditions. In matters of your health
care, we recommend that you consult a qualified health practitioner and
not attempt to self-treat based on information in this book.

© 1993 Rosita Arvigo and Michael Balick
All rights reserved. No part of this book may be reproduced in any form or by
any electronic or mechanical means including informationstorage and retrieval
systems without permission in writing from the publisher, except by a reviewer
who may quote brief passages in review.

First Edition December 1993
Printed in the United States of America

ISBN 0-914955-13-6
Library of Congress #93-80280

Published in 1993 by
Lotus Press / Box 325 / Twin Lakes, WI 53181

Printed on recycled paper with soy ink.

DEDICATED TO

THE TRADITIONAL HEALERS OF BELIZE

AND THEIR FOREBEARERS . . .

AND TO THE FUTURE GENERATIONS THAT

WILL LEARN AND TEACH THEIR WISDOM

TABLE OF CONTENTS

FOREWORD

I first learned of Rosita Arvigo and Michael Balick from a news segment about their work in the rainforests of Belize. I recognized that we shared an interest in preserving the cultural diversity of indigenous people and a sense that, as the rainforests are lost, so are the cultures that thrive within them. Their stories, songs, traditions, and knowledge are no longer practiced and passed on to successive generations when the environment in which they survive is destroyed. This loss is one of the great tragedies of our time, and one that is not fully appreciated. In many ways, the work in this book parallels my own in its purpose, the preservation of music and the cultures that produce it.

In devoting themselves to the study of the identification and uses of medicinal plants by the healers of Belize, Drs. Arvigo and Balick open a door for us into the sacred world of shamans, traditional healers who know that the rainforest holds within its grasp all the ingredients that have sustained it and its people. The authors bring this traditional knowledge to the attention of scientists, medical practitioners, and the world at large. By cataloging these plants and their uses for this book, they amplify, through the modern media, the voices of those who have not been heard. The publication of information that had previously been passed on only through oral tradition places value on, and draws attention to, that knowledge. In recognizing the value of this information to our own lives, we send a message to the people of the rainforest that their knowledge is important to us and that its loss would be a devastating loss for all humankind.

In their book and through their work, Drs. Arvigo and Balick light the fires and carry the torch toward preservation of the rainforests and the indigenous cultures that exist within them. There is a chance for us to do something before these cultures vanish, and people like Drs. Arvigo and Balick are leading the way. I hope you will enjoy this glimpse of their journey as much as I have.

Mickey Hart
October 1993

ACKNOWLEDGEMENTS

We have been privileged to study with a number of gifted and knowledgeable traditional healers through our work with the Belize Ethnobotany Project. This book is the beneficiary of information generously taught us by numerous individuals in the traditional healing community in Belize, representing the diverse cultural heritage to be found within this country's borders. We are especially grateful to the following: Doña Juana Cuc and Sr. Antonio Cuc of San Antonio, Cayo, patriarchs who have cared for many generations using traditional plant remedies; Miss Barbara Fernandez of Belize City, who has an herb shop in the Belize City market that is well known and respected throughout the country and who has authored *Medicine Woman: The Herbal Tradition of Belize*, a book on medicinal herbs; Mr. Thomas Green, of the Cayo District, who learned his trade in the chicle, rubber, and mahogany camps, and is an accomplished canoe craftsman as well; Mr. Winston Harris, of Cristo Rey, Cayo District, known as a master of jungle survival (bushmaster), as well as a snake bite healer; Don Eligio Panti, originally from the Peten of Guatemala, now resident of San Antonio, Cayo District, who is the most famous of all traditional healers in Belize and, indeed, throughout much of Central America (although his father was an infamous practitioner of black magic, Don Eligio occupies the highest level of Mayan healing, that of doctor-priest); Mr. Andrew Ramcharan, Ranchito, Corozal District, known as the most accomplished snake bite healer in all of the north of Belize, a crucial skill in an area covered with sugar cane fields that harbor many snakes; Miss Hortense Robinson, of Ladyville, Belize District, who has been a midwife for over 50 years, and works as a general practitioner specializing in ailments of women and children; Mr. Polo Romero, an accomplished snake doctor, bushmaster and officer of the Belize Association of Traditional Healers, who learned his craft while working in rubber, mahogany, and chicle camps; and Doña Juana Xix, of Sukkotz Village, Cayo District, who is a primary health care specialist and midwife to residents of many of the surrounding villages. It is primarily to these great healers that we owe our thanks.

This book and, indeed, all of our work in Belize has been blessed with the kindness and support of many others in Belize, as well. Lou Nicolait of The Belize Environmental Center has been a loyal friend and a source of inspiration and strength. The Belize Forestry Department has encouraged us in many ways, and for this we thank Richard Belisle, Earl Green, Jackie Herrera, and Oscar Rosado. The Belize College of Agriculture, Central Farms has shared a strong interest in our work, and we particularly appreciate the collaboration of Carol August, John Link, and Hugh O'Brien. Sharon Matola has imparted to us her strong sense of conservation and has helped us develop a paradigm for ethnobotanical conservation in the Belizean context. At the U.S. Agency for International Development Mission to Belize, Jeffrey

Allen, Paul Bisek, Mosina Jordan, George Like, and Barbara Sandoval have been enthusiastic in their support of our work. Bob Jones of Eva's Restaurant in San Ignacio, Cayo, has been a consistent friend who has always been interested in our endeavors.

At The New York Botanical Garden, numerous individuals have contributed in many ways to this effort. Sincere thanks go to Cathy Alexander, Miguel Alexiades, Rupert Barneby, Hans Beck, Brian Boom, John Brown, Douglas Daly, Enrique Forereo, Sandi Frank, Rosemarie Garipoli, James Hester, Marianne Holden, Jackie Kallunki, Gregory Long, Zoë Marchal, Michael Nee, Ann Rumsey, Carol Salera, and, especially, to the staffs of the Herbarium and Library, as well as to the botanists of the Institute of Systematic Botany and their fellow systematists around the world who have provided the identifications for the plants on which this book is based. We are grateful to Elizabeth Pecchia for her meticulous and caring preparation of this manuscript and to Jan Wassmer Stevenson for her sensitive and critical reading of it in its later stages. Special thanks are due our colleague Willa Capraro for her dedication to the production of this book. Her editorial assistance and compilation of the glossary, index, and bibliography are especially appreciated. The preparation of camera-ready copy of any publication requires a meticulous eye and caring attitude, and we appreciate Willa's efforts in seeing this through to completion.

We are grateful for the enthusiastic support of our field assistants, who work in the collecting and pressing of the voucher and bulk collections. Since 1987, these have included Pablo Cocom, Rolando Cocom, Garfield Ramcharan, John Woodland, Eddy Xix, and Manolo Xix. Other participants in our field work have been Louis Connick, William Farrell, Christian Heckert, Jay Holmes, Marshall Horwitz, Susan Horwitz, Jean Kadel, Irene Kendall, Heather McCargo, Roberto Melendez, Antonio Morales, Andrew Reed, Deborah Sampson-Ripley, David Sostman, and Katy Valk.

We are particularly grateful to Norman Farnsworth, Charlotte Gyllenhaal-Huft, and Ruth Quimby of the University of Illinois at Chicago who have provided us with NAPRALERT searches. At Shaman Pharmaceuticals, Steven King and Alondra Oubré were generous in supplying us with computer-generated literature searches about Belizean plants, as were Tom Carlson and Carey Jackson who gave us their professional critiques of the medical terms in our glossary. James Duke of the United States Department of Agriculture supplied us with an extensive list of chemicals contained within these plants, a list of compounds so detailed that they will be issued as a supplement to this volume. Ann Bradburn of Tulane University offered early guidance in our work. Mark Blumenthal's thoughtful review of the manuscript is much appreciated.

We have received support for our endeavors in Belize from a coalition of philanthropic agencies and individuals who felt that our work could make a difference. For this, we owe a debt of gratitude that can never be repaid, and we hope that our project contributions are worthy of that support. Our gratitude is extended to The U.S. National Institutes of Health/National Cancer Institute, The U.S. Agency for International Development, The Rockefeller Foundation, The Metropolitan Life Insurance Foundation, The Overbrook Foundation, The Edward John Noble Foundation, The Philecology Trust, The Rex Foundation, The John and Catherine T. MacArthur Foundation, The Nathan Cummings Foundation, as well as to individual contributors Kathy Gallagher, Mary R. Kemmerer, Bruce McCowan, and Mary R. Morgan. Special thanks go to Diana Landreth Altschul, Adam Cummings, and Mickey Hart for believing in us from the very beginning.

We are also grateful to our critics, who, knowingly or not, have helped us navigate in increasingly complex waters and make mid-course changes when appropriate. It is only through these trials and errors that we can hope to develop the project philosophies and technologies that could be of use to others elsewhere.

Santosh Krinsky and his colleagues at Lotus Press, in particular, Nirankar Agarwal and Navaja Llope, have been most helpful and patient with us during the preparation of this book.

Very, very special thanks go to Gregory Shropshire who has been our friend and partner in the field and in the birth of The Ix Chel Tropical Research Foundation and The Belize Ethnobotany Project. For Greg, nothing is ever impossible.

Rosita Arvigo, D.N.
Michael Balick, Ph.D.

INTRODUCTION

BACKGROUND

Belize is a country of great resources, both physical and spiritual. Strengthened by the heterogeneity of nine distinct cultural and ethnic groups to be found within her borders, Belize is a land of great natural beauty. In contrast to many of her neighbors in Central America and the Caribbean, Belize has a wealth of forest lands and a system of protected forest reserves which, although fragile, are evidence of the country's strong commitment to conservation of its natural resources.

Unfortunately, knowledge about the utility of native plants, particularly as medicines, that has been refined over scores of generations is probably in greater danger of extinction at the present time than are the plant resources. Thousands of years ago, the native peoples of Central America had great centers of learning, including medical schools that taught the role of plants in health care. With the decline of these civilizations, and the arrival of the Spanish Conquistadors, many cultural practices, including the teaching of this information, declined or were banned entirely. Among the losses were the great books (codexes) of the Maya, which contained a wealth of knowledge about the uses of plants in medicine and which were burned by the Spanish. Additionally, intergenerational transmission of information about useful plants shifted from a written to an oral tradition. For example, mother would take daughter into the forest and, once out of earshot of the Spanish, teach her about childbirth and the plants that could be used to help ease the pain of labor. Father would take son into a cave and teach him about the Mayan spirits, and about the ceremonial uses of plants and the holy rituals. Such patterns are evident for other indigenous cultures, as well.

Sadly, modern times have led to the further loss of a great deal of information about plant use, known as ethnobotanical information, throughout the world. Today, in Belize, it is common to hear that "while grandfather knew a lot about healing plants, he only taught my father a little, and I am more interested in modern life and, therefore, didn't pay much attention to the subject while I was growing up." It is the work of the ethnobotanist to chronicle this information, to document the remnants of what once existed, and to make it freely available to all who wish it, including future generations.

The authors of this volume were introduced to each other through a newspaper clipping sent to Dr. Arvigo about the work of Dr. Balick. Through correspondence and during our first face to face conversation, we realized that we shared many common goals in the field of ethnobotany and traditional medicine. Thus, in 1987, The Belize Ethnobotany Project was born, a decade-long survey of the ethnobotanical wealth of Belize, designed to record much of the often-endangered information about plants used as medicines, foods, and fiber; in construction and agriculture; during religious ceremonies; and as part of spiritual beliefs. The project has resulted in the creation of The Ix Chel Tropical Research Foundation, a non-governmental organization based in the Cayo District, dedicated to traditional medicine, ethnobotanical studies, Belizean culture, and rainforest conservation. It has also helped in the formation of The Belize Association of Traditional Healers and Terra Nova Rainforest Reserve, an extractive reserve for medicinal plants officially established on June 24, 1993.

METHODOLOGY AND PURPOSE

It is beyond the scope of this book to describe the complete methodology involved in ethnobotanical investigation, but we believe that a summary will be of interest to the reader. Beginning in 1987 and working with a number of Belizean traditional medical practitioners, we began to collect and document the use of plant ethnomedicines. Detailed information on use was collected and herbarium specimens that serve as vouchers for the information were made. The herbarium specimens (plants pressed between newspapers) were dried at low heat in an oven. In this way, the dried stems, leaves, fruits, flowers, etc. that comprise the herbarium specimen are preserved and can be affixed to a large sheet of rag bond paper. This ensures that the individual specimen, if properly curated, will last hundreds of years. Some 2,800 specimens were collected in all; each was then sent out to a plant systematist, over one hundred of whom assisted us, to verify its identity and obtain its most current scientific name. The plants, collected in duplicate series of 4-6, were then distributed to herbaria both in Belize and in the U.S. to serve as a permanent record of this study. In Belize, the specimens are to be found at the Belize College of Agriculture, Central Farms, and the Forestry Department Herbarium in Belmopan. Specimen sets are on deposit at The New York Botanical Garden, the Smithsonian Institution, and the Gray Herbarium of Harvard University, while duplicate sets have been distributed to taxonomic specialists in exchange for their opinions. Following the identification of the plants, we produced descriptions of each of the species discussed in this book, along with a report on its local use in traditional medicine. We then added information on common names, in some cases including notes on folklore. Following this, we searched through the literature to gather what was known about the pharmacology and chemistry of each of the different species. This search was greatly aided by the use of the NAPRALERT (Natural Products Alert) data base system developed by the staff of the University of Illinois at Chicago. Finally, a black and white illustration was prepared by artist Laura Evans for each of the species discussed.

Not infrequently, we have been asked why the process from specimen collection to publication of the results takes so many years. The coordination of specimen-related activities, including their collection, shipment, and identification by numerous taxonomic specialists at institutions around the world, in itself took several years to accomplish. Following this, the lengthy process of researching and writing the book could commence, in between field trips, lectures, and other activities. Thus, we are grateful for the continuing patience of our supporters and many colleagues, especially the traditional healers, with whom we have worked year after year and who only now will see the written results of these labors.

The process of collecting ethnobotanical data from individuals can be the most rewarding aspect of our fieldwork. The traditional healers and bushmasters are a rare breed of individuals who have usually overcome great personal hardships and major illnesses of their own to gain the acquired knowledge of medicinal plants. Over the years, we have had an opportunity to observe those personality traits which epitomize the traditional healers of Belize: tremendous self-confidence, a great sense of humor, a strong spiritual foundation, an abiding humility, a great respect for the natural world and its ability to sustain life, and a sense of caring more for the welfare of others than for their own. It is always an awesome and inspiring experience to be in their presence, and a humbling one to gain their love and confidence.

The ethnobotanist must approach traditional healers or bushmasters with the utmost sensitivity, respecting their cultural heritage and limitations of age, health, and time. All too often researchers arrive unannounced at the home or clinic of a healer bearing machines, batteries, lights, collection equipment, cameras, and notebooks poised for action, only to close the door they came to open. A better methodology is to seek an introduction, make several visits to sit and chat and, within that exchange, explain the purpose of the research work and what role the traditional healer would play. Issues of intellectual property rights and compensation must be acknowledged and discussed. It must be made clear as to how the healer would receive just recognition for his or her contribution. Some healers do not wish to share their information -- their decision should be respected and accepted gracefully, as there are usually valid reasons behind it.

Most traditional healers are thrilled to know that they can help to pass the torch of healing to another generation. They are deeply concerned that the young people of today care little about healing plants and "old-fashioned" ways. From every corner of the globe, we learn that the fires of traditional healing are now, in the twentieth century, down to a mere bed of embers and faintly glowing coals. If we do not place fresh fuel on this bed of embers and continue to blow on the coals from generation to generation, the fire may become extinguished.

So, what our project and this book are about is helping to keep that fire -- that torch -- burning brightly. This book is a part of that effort and represents a collaboration among traditional healers, biological scientists, and alternative physicians, each of whom has attempted to place a substantial log on this bed of coals.

SCOPE OF BOOK

It was our intention to produce an easily readable manual that would chronicle the information so generously provided to us over the last several years. In addition to serving as a registry of cultural information concerning Belizean plants, the book is also designed to be used in the local classroom, amongst the communities of traditional healers and environmentalists, and for general background on the ethnobotany of Central America. It is our intention that a portion of the revenues generated by the sales of this book will help subsidize its distribution in some of these areas. Perhaps, in so doing, we will be able to express our gratitude to the traditional healers with whom we have worked, as well as to the people of Belize who have been so friendly and receptive to our endeavors.

Caveats

It must be emphasized that this book is not intended to serve as a manual for self-medication, or as a substitute for qualified medical advice. The Caribbean pharmacopoeias produced through the well known TRAMIL program fall much closer to this goal with their recommendations of species to be used, to be avoided, and those to be further investigated. For the most part, the research results that we report here are intended to give an overview of the pharmacological properties of Belizean plants and certainly not to endorse any particular utilization by humans. It should be made clear that perceived biological activity in animal or *in vitro* systems very often has little correlation with what could be expected in human clinical results. Although we have included information on specific toxic properties of some plants commonly used in Belize in the section on "research results," the absence of such information for a particular plant should not be construed to mean that the plant has no harmful properties.

Organization of text and illustrations

In order to make access to the information in this book as easy as possible for the reader, we have opted to use the English common name for each plant as the primary means of identification. This name has been printed in **bold and capitalized** typeface at the top of each page and the plants have been arranged alphabetically according to these names. In some cases, we felt that a non-English name would be more recognizable and, so, it became the primary name; a letter code following the name identifies its origin (see below for explanation of letter code). When known to us, other local names have also been listed beneath the primary name; again, a letter code designates the origin of each of these local names, e.g., (E) for English; (S) for Spanish; (M) for Maya -- usually Mopan Maya; (C) for Creole. The abbreviation "Men." is used to designate Mennonite origin.

Scientific name: This is a species name, known as a binomial because it always consists of two words: the first word denotes the genus, which may contain one or more species, while the second word is the specific epithet and is particular to the species. Each word in the binomial is either of Latin origin or has been given a Latinized form and has been printed in *italics*. The species name is followed by a letter or name indicating the author(s), i.e., the person or persons who described the species. When an author's name has been abbreviated, this is by convention.

Plant family: There are various systems for grouping plant species into families. We have used the classification system proposed by the late Dr. Arthur Cronquist in *An Integrated System of Classification of Flowering Plants.* (New York: Columbia University Press, 1981.)

Description: This is a simple description of the plant as it appears in the field, highlighting those characteristics which we feel will be most obvious and, therefore, useful to the reader. It is usually a modification of the descriptions which appear in selected parts of the scientific journal *Fieldiana: Botany* (Flora of Guatemala, Volume 24, Parts I-XII, 1946-1970; Ferns and Fern Allies of Guatemala, New Series, #6, Part II: Polypodiaceae, 1981).

Habitat: This indicates the most common areas in which the plant is to be found, and whether it occurs in the wild or in cultivation.

Traditional uses: This is a compilation of specific information from the following sources -- (1) reports from healers and/or (2) personal observations of plant use in Belize. These are not recommendations for their use, however, as we recognize that plant usage is quite different depending upon the background of the individual healer. In fact, universal agreement about much of the plant material (especially with respect to dosage and preparation) is rare. On the other hand, we have found a number of plants that are known by virtually everyone and that have many universally known uses -- we refer to these as "powerful plants."

Research results: For the most part, these are the results of laboratory research. In some cases (e.g., Kingsbury 1964), instances of direct observations are also cited. Wherever we have included research results in the text, we have also indicated the literature in which the findings have been reported. We cannot stress too strongly that this section is _not_ intended as a recommendation to use a plant in any particular way. *Please refer to the "Caveats" above for more information about this section.*

Illustrations: Each verbal discussion of a plant is accompanied by a drawing which illustrates one or more key features useful in the field identification of the plant.

Other related publications

This book is the second major publication arising from the Belize Ethnobotany Project through The Ix Chel Tropical Research Foundation and The New York Botanical Garden Institute of Economic Botany. The first, which appeared in 1991, is "Useful Plants of the Mundo Maya -- A Colouring Book," by Dr. Rosita Arvigo, illustrated by Tessa Fairweather. Other publications to be produced through The Belize Ethnobotany Project include "A Checklist of the Flowering Plants and Ferns of Belize, with Annotations on Common Names and Uses," as well as a more comprehensive volume containing detailed descriptions and use data on the ca. 1,000 species we have recorded in Belize that are consumed as food, or utilized for construction, fiber, oil, resin, medicine, or for spiritual purposes. This volume, "Messages from the Gods -- The Ethnobotanical Wealth of Belize," will also have much more detailed chapters on the economic value of the non-timber forest products of Belize, pharmacological data from our National Cancer Institute-sponsored collection program carried out in collaboration with the Forestry Department and Belize Environmental Center, chapters on local disease concepts and beliefs, and detailed information on other aspects of the work of the individual healers. As we have a particular interest in the Arecaceae, we are also planning a volume on the palms of Belize and their uses. Finally, a computerized data base containing all of the information collected during the field expeditions and in subsequent follow-up studies with traditional healers will be available. We hope that this will be housed at both the Forestry Department and Belize Environmental Center.

ETHNOBOTANY AND INTELLECTUAL PROPERTY RIGHTS

It is our strong feeling that all of the information that has been provided us should be freely shared with those who wish to use it for the public good, and be chronicled for future generations. We also believe that the information should be available to all parties simultaneously, and not solely to those who wish to use it for their own personal gain or political agenda. However, like it or not, politics is an inseparable aspect of scientific research, especially in areas such as intellectual property rights. Unfortunately, some traditional healers and others have been involved in anthropological, ethnobotanical, pharmacological or other studies, either local or international, with little idea of the potential impact of their contributions and with no mechanism for them, their communities, or their countries to benefit from new discoveries or applications of their knowledge. To address this situation, we have insisted on working only with reputable individuals, both inside of Belize and elsewhere, toward the goals of The Belize Ethnobotany Project. In a recent position paper by The Belize Association of Traditional Healers, the suggestion was made that benefits arising from these types of studies be assigned to the community of traditional healers. Our work with the U.S. National Cancer Institute, a non-profit agency, provides for such benefits to the healers' community. However, those benefits may be a decade or more away, and so we have put other mechanisms in place for more immediate benefits. For example, this project has helped to build an herbarium reference collection at the Belize College of Agriculture and at the Belize Forestry Department, which will not only improve scientific information, but may also help to promote respect for the teachings of these healers within their own nations. Additionally, a portion of the profits from the sale of this book will go to help both the healers who worked with us to achieve their own personal goals, such as the construction of clinics, as well as to the Belize Association of Traditional Healers to help it to further enhance traditional healing in Belize. A rebirth of interest in traditional healing, through education, agricultural trials with native plants, seminars and lectures to the lay public, interaction with medical professionals, and ecological- and scientific-based tourism will help create employment opportunities and contribute to the economic development of the area. We also expect that this rebirth of interest will help rekindle respect for the knowledge of the elders in the community and foster renewed interest in the traditional culture. We would welcome additional suggestions from the readers as to ways in which practitioners can realize increased benefits from their work.

GLOSSARY

The following terms have been paraphrased or adapted from a variety of sources, including the references listed at the end of this section and our personal observations on their use in Belize.

abortifacient, abortive. Substance or action that induces abortion.

abscess. A collection of pus anywhere in or on the body.

alimentary tract. The digestive system.

amoebas. Microscopic one-celled animals that live in soil or water, but can become parasitic in humans.

analgesic activity. Ability to stop or reduce pain.

anemia. Reduction of red cells in the blood; there are many causes of anemia and the treatment differs with each cause.

anesthetic activity. Total or partial loss of sensation. If administered regionally or locally, the patient remains conscious; if administered generally, the patient loses consciousness.

annual. An herbaceous plant that dies down at the end of each growing season.

antiascariasis activity. Inhibiting the growth of parasitic intestinal worms in the nematode genus *Ascaris*.

antibacterial activity. Inhibiting the growth of bacteria.

anticonvulsant activity. Reducing or stopping convulsions.

antidote. That which counteracts the effects of a poisonous substance.

antiestrogenic effect. Ability to counteract the effects of the female hormone estrogen.

antifertility agent. Interfering with fertilization (i.e., reproduction) or the implantation of an embryo into the uterine wall.

antifungal activity. Ability to interfere with the growth of fungal infections.

antihemorrhagic activity. Ability to reduce or stop bleeding. *See also* hemorrhage.

antihyperglycemic activity. Ability to lower an abnormally high level of blood sugar (glucose).

anti-inflammatory activity. Reduces or stops inflammation. *See also* inflammation.

antimalarial activity. Ability to suppress or kill the *Plasmodium* parasite that causes malaria. *See also* malaria.

antiparasitic activity. Ability to suppress or kill parasites. *See also* parasite.

antischistosomal activity. Ability to suppress or kill a fresh water *Schistosoma* parasite, which is transmitted by snails.

antispasmodic activity. Ability to reduce or stop spasms.

antituberculosis activity. Ability to suppress or kill the *Mycobacterium tuberculosis* bacterium that causes tuberculosis.

antiulcer activity. Preventing or lessening the development of ulcers. *See also* ulcer.

antiviral activity. Ability to suppress or kill viruses.

antiyeast activity. Ability to suppress or kill yeast (a group of fungi).

arthritis. Inflammation of the joint(s). Symptoms often include swelling, pain, redness, heat, and tissue structural changes.

ascaricidal activity. Ability to suppress or kill intestinal worms in the genus *Ascaris*.

asthma. Difficult and sometimes painful breathing and wheezing, due to spasms or constriction of bronchial passages.

astringent. Having ability to constrict tissues, stop secretion, or control bleeding.

atole. A soft drink made from corn (maize) flour. (Spanish)

axil (of leaf). The upper angle formed by the joining of a leaf to a stem.

bajo. Local Spanish name for steam bath. Used extensively for muscle pain, paralysis, swelling, and water retention in people of all ages. *See also* herbal bathing.

barbs. Sharp outgrowths on plant, usually ending with a reflexed hook (as in a fishing hook).

berry. A type of fruit characterized by a fleshy or juicy pulp in which the seeds are embedded.

biliousness. A liver condition in which bile builds up, causing such symptoms as constipation, headache, loss of appetite, vomiting, and irritability.

bipinnate; twice-pinnate. A compound leaf in which the main stem branches once and the leaflets on the secondary stem are divided into segments. *See also* pinnate.

boil. An inflammation occurring under the top layer of skin caused by a localized bacterial infection in a hair follicle.

bract. A modified leaf that originates at the base of a flower or flower cluster. Its function is variable and includes showiness (as in Poinsettia), protection (as in bud scales), etc.

bronchitis. Inflammation of the bronchial passages.

bulb. A short underground bud consisting of a vertical conical stem with several thickened, overlapping storage leaves attached to its base. Examples include members of the lily and onion families.

bushmaster. An individual who spends a considerable amount of time in the forest and is considered highly knowledgeable about it and the uses of forest plants and animals.

calyx. The collective term used for all of the sepals on a flower; the outermost whorl of a flower.

GLOSSARY

cancer. The local Spanish term used for an ailment characterized by severe, weeping, open wounds that are chronic, spreading, and difficult to heal. This concept of cancer is quite different from that of conventional (Western) medicine.

capsule. A type of dry fruit characterized by having two or more sections which split open at maturity to release seeds.

carcinogenic activity. Ability to cause cancer as understood by conventional (Western) medical practitioners; for example, promoting tumor growth.

cardiac depressant activity. Causing a decrease in heart function, specifically in the rate of heartbeat and the ability of the heart muscles to contract.

cardiotoxic activity. Poisonous to the heart.

cataracts. A condition of the eyes in which the lens and/or capsule around the lens becomes cloudy or opaque.

catarrh, infantile. An inflammation of the mucous membranes in the nose and throat of infants, causing an increased flow of mucous secretions.

chiclero. The Spanish word for a gatherer of latex from the Sapodilla tree (known as "chicle") which formed the base for commercial chewing gum before synthetic chewing gum replaced it in the 1930's. *Chicleros* were considered excellent bushmasters with an extensive knowledge of useful plants.

coagulant activity. Ability to stop bleeding.

colic, infantile. Condition occurring in first few months of infant's life, involving pain-causing intestinal spasms; often attributed to gassiness.

colitis. A condition of the colon (large intestine) in which it becomes inflamed.

congested blood. A perceived increase in the amount of blood that is normally found in any body part. The local Spanish term for this is *pasmo.*

conjunctivitis. Inflammation of the mucous membranes lining the eyeball and eyelid.

constrict. To bind, squeeze, or make narrow, as with blood vessels, heart muscles, etc.

Creole. Individuals having some degree of African ancestry and speaking the local English Creole dialect.

cultivated. Not growing wild; planted and grown for human use. An example would be food crops.

cytotoxic activity. Ability to destroy cells.

deciduous. Falling off, as leaves do at the end of a growing season; opposite of evergreen.

decoction. A liquid preparation made by boiling plant parts in water.

dementia. Diminished mental capacity. May take a variety of forms including depression, delusions, memory loss, erratic or inappropriate behavior, etc.

dermatitis, contact. Inflammation of the skin arising from "contact with an irritating substance." Common symptoms include redness and itching.

dilate. To spread, enlarge, expand, or stretch a hollow organ or opening.

diuretic. A treatment which increases urination.

drupe. A type of fruit characterized by having an outer "skin," surrounding a soft pulp, with a hard, stony "pit" in the center. (Quotes reflect non-botanical terms commonly applied to these parts.)

dysentery. Intestinal disease involving inflammation of the intestinal mucous membranes and caused by invasive agents such as amoebas and certain bacteria and parasites. Common symptoms include diarrhea with blood and sometimes with mucus. Dysentery is often accompanied by intestinal spasms and abdominal pain.

edema. "An accumulation of an excessive amount of watery fluid in cells, tissues, or serous cavities" in the body. Edema may result in a swollen limb.

ellipsoidal. Having an elliptical form, somewhat like a circle that has been elongated. *See also* elliptical.

elliptical. Broadest in the middle and narrowing at both ends.

embryotoxic effect. Having a poisonous effect on an organism in the embryonic stages of development.

emollient. Something that softens or soothes the part of the body to which it is applied. Examples include body lotions and oils, petroleum jelly.

empacho. Local Spanish word for an intestinal obstruction.

emphysema. A condition of the lungs, in which the small air sacs of the lungs (alveoli) are damaged. The most common symtom is difficulty in breathing; frequent coughing may also occur.

endosperm. The tissue in seeds of flowering plants which surrounds and provides food for the embryo. In coconuts, the endosperm of an immature seed is a milky liquid which becomes jelly-like and finally hard as the seed matures.

ensalmos. Local Spanish word for healing prayers.

envy. Also known locally as *envidia* (in Spanish). This is a common spiritual ailment in Belize caused by a neighbor or companion who daily looks upon another's life with envy and jealousy, thereby causing the object of the envy to become ill with any of a wide range of symptoms such as weakness, confusion, indigestion, and fear, as well as lack of incentive and feelings of hopelessness.

epiphytic. A plant that uses another plant as a substrate without taking nutrients from it (i.e., not parasitic). For example, many bromeliads are epiphytic.

erect. Standing upright, as an upright stem; opposite of prostrate.

evil. This is a spiritual disease which is also known locally as *maldad* and *obeah*. It is believed to be caused by evil spirits. Symptoms are varied and include nightmares, malaise, bad luck, sores, itching skin, indigestion, errant voices, unexplainable fear, and great anxiety.

evil eye. Also known locally as the "hot eye," the "bad eye," and the "eye." Many people throughout Central America believe that certain people can cause inanimate objects to break, and people to become ill as a result of their envious glances.

expectorant. Loosens mucus in throat or lungs, enabling patient to cough it up and expel it.

extravasations. The movement of fluids from their containing vessels (such as, blood vessels, lymph nodes) to the surrounding tissue, as in the formation of a bruise by the accumulation of blood in the tissue.

exudes. Flows or oozes out of. For example, the latex of the chicle tree will flow out of the tree when the bark is cut, while resin will ooze from cut pine bark.

fern. One of the spore-bearing (as opposed to flowering) vascular plants. Ferns display a variety of growth habits in a variety of habitats. Examples include epiphytic, aquatic, and terrestrial forms; tree height versus tiny; etc.

fever. A rise in body temperature above the level considered normal for an individual.

filament. The stalklike part of a flower that supports the pollen-bearing anther.

flatulence. Gassiness in the stomach and intestines.

forest, primary. Forest that has not been cut or otherwise disturbed.

forest margins. The outer edges of a forested area.

forest, secondary. Forest that has regenerated after a disturbance of some sort, whether natural (as after lightening-caused fire) or man-made (as after lumbering or slash and burn cultivation).

galactagogue effect. Acting to bring on the flow of mother's milk.

gastric ulcer. An ulceration of the lining of the stomach. *See also* ulcer.

Garífuna. Also known as "Caribs," these are descendents of black Hondurans who immigrated to Belize during the first half of the 19th century. Many now live in the southern coastal areas; they have retained a distinctive language and culture.

gastritis. Stomach inflammation. Typical symptoms include pain, burning sensation, nausea, and sometimes vomiting.

germination inhibition in plants. Ability to prevent a seed from sprouting.

glabrous. Smooth; without hair.

glaucous. Having a waxy, whitish, or greyish "bloom" which can be rubbed off.

globose. Round, like a globe or ball.

glochids. Small, hair-like spines found on certain cacti such as *Opuntia*.

gonorrhea. A contagious disease that is caused by the *Neisseria gonorrhoeae* bacteria and is transmitted through sexual contact. The disease typically affects the mucous membranes of the genitalia. Symptoms include discharge from the urethra and pain on urination. If not treated, infection may spread to joints, heart, and other organs.

handful; double handful. Term designating the amount of herbs to use in a given formula. This is a traditional measurement which allows each person to receive a metered dose: one handful is the amount that fits into one cupped palm; a double handful is the amount that can be held in two hands that are cupped together.

head (of a flower). Tight terminal cluster of florets on short or no stalks, as seen in members of the aster family.

heat. A local concept, also referred to in Spanish as *calor*, that includes various physical conditions characterized by fever, rashes, perspiration, restlessness, and swelling. **Cold** (*frieldad* in Spanish), on the other hand, encompasses a range of physical ailments primarily characterized by cramping, spasms, paralysis, menstrual cramps, infertility in both men and women, mucus discharge, congestion, and blockage of blood circulation.

hemorrhage. Excessive bleeding; may be too heavy a flow or bleeding where there should be none.

hepatitis. A condition in which the liver becomes inflamed. Common symptoms include jaundice (a yellowing of the skin), fever, and diarrhea.

hepatotoxic activity. Ability to injure liver cells.

herb; herbaceous. Non-woody plant that dies down to the ground at the end of each growing season.

herbal bathing. An integral part of Mayan traditional healing, this is used for a variety of ailments, but especially for skin conditions, muscle spasms, backache, nervous disorders, insomnia, bruises, and swellings. All children's ailments receive a series of herbal baths. The baths are made with combinations of medicinal leaves mixed into formulas to suit age, sex, and symptoms. *See also bajo.*

GLOSSARY

hypertensive activity. Having effect of increasing blood pressure above a level considered normal.
hypoglycemic activity. Having effect of lowering blood sugar (glucose level).
hypotensive activity. Having effect of lowering blood pressure.
hypothermic activity. Having effect of lowering body temperature.

impotency (in males). Inability to sustain erection of the penis.
indigestion. Digestion that has not been completed and which may produce gassiness, belching, heartburn, pain, or nausea.
inflammation (general). The reaction of tissue to physical or chemical injury or to an infection. The most common symptoms include pain, heat, redness, swelling, and reduced mobility.
inflorescence. Term applied to the arrangement of flowers on a stem or branch. There are several different types of inflorescences.
insecticidal activity. Ability to kill insects.
insomnia. A consistent pattern in which an individual is unable to fall or remain asleep.
irritación. The local Spanish word for an infantile disease characterized by fever, swollen belly, cold hands and feet, perspiration, and diarrhea.

Kekchi. *See* Maya.

lanceolate (leaf). Long and narrow, wider above the base and narrowing toward the tip.
larvae. An immature stage in the life cycle of some insects. At this stage, the insect usually appears worm- or grub-like; for example, a caterpillar.
latex. A runny and/or sticky substance that is found in specialized conductive canals (called laticifers) in many plants; it may flow or ooze out when the plant is cut into or broken. Though chemically and structurally different from resin, both substances may appear the same and all latexes contain some degree of resin. (For example, chicle and rubber, both latexes, contain 40% and 3% resin, respectively.) *See also* resin.
laxative. Induces bowel movement; used to counteract constipation.
leaflets. The segments of a compound leaf.
legume. A member of the pea (Fabaceae) family. Its characteristic fruit is dry and splits along two sutures to release seeds.
leukorrhea. A discharge of white or yellowish fluid from the vaginal area.
lobe. An indented segment (usually rounded) of a leaf or flower.

malaise. A vague or generalized feeling of being unwell or uncomfortable.

malaria. A disease of the red blood cells in which a protozoa (the *Plasmodium* parasite) is transmitted to the blood stream via the bite of the *Anopheles* mosquito (usual means of transmission) or some other means, such as blood transfusion.

margins. Edges, as of leaves or forests.

mastitis. Breast inflammation.

Maya. The collective term used locally to designate people of three Mayan groups: the **Mopan**, the **Yucatec**, and the **Kekchí**.

Mennonite. A member of a religious order of Protestant Christians.

menses. A woman's monthly "period"; menstruation.

molluscicidal activity. Ability to kill molluscs (such as snails) which often parasitize other organisms.

Mopan. *See* Maya.

muscle (smooth) relaxant activity. Having effect of relaxing the involuntary muscles that are found usually in internal organs such as the digestive and respiratory systems.

mutagenic. Having ability to cause mutations.

necrosis. The death of an area of cells, tissue, or bone.

nephrotoxic activity. Ability to injure kidney cells.

neuralgia. Pain occurring "along the course or distribution of a nerve."

oblong (leaf shape). Longer than broad, with sides that are nearly parallel.

obovate (leaf shape). Somewhat in the shape of an egg, but broadest above the middle.

ovoid (leaf shape). Egg-shaped.

palmate (leaf arrangement). Having three or more leaves or leaf segments arranged so that they radiate outward from a central point, like the fingers of a hand.

panacea. A remedy that is viewed as being able to cure all ailments.

panicle. An infloresence in the form of a branching cluster of flowers.

parasite. An organism that lives on or in another organism (known as the host) and which depends upon the host organism to meet its nutritional needs. A **plant parasite** might obtain water, or nutrients, or both from its plant host. An **intestinal parasite** (such as a worm) invades the intestinal tract of its animal host.

pasmo. The local Spanish word for congested blood: a perceived increase in the amount of blood that is normally found in any body part.

perennial. A plant that lives three or more years and, usually, flowers each year.

pesticide. Used to kill pests, including weeds, rodents, and insects.

petiole (of leaf). The stem or stalk of a simple leaf; the main stem or stalk of a compound leaf (but not of the leaflets).

phytophotodermatitis. An inflammation of the skin caused by contact with a plant substance (for example, the oil of citrus) in the presence of sunlight.

photosensitivity. Sensitivity to light.

piles. Hemorrhoids; swollen blood vessels in the rectum.

pinna (singular); pinnae (plural). The leaflets or segments of a pinnately compound leaf, as in ferns and palms.

pinnate; pinnately-compound. Having a blade divided into segments or leaflets that are arranged along either side of a single unbranched stalk. In **bipinnate** or **twice-pinnate** leaves, the main stalk is branched once so that the leaflets are further divided into segments.

pistillate (flower). Having only the female reproductive parts (pistils).

pleurisy. An inflammation of the mucous membranes around the lungs.

pod. A type of dry fruit which splits along two sutures to release seeds, typical of the pea (Fabaceae) family.

postoperative. Following surgery.

postpartum. Following childbirth.

poultice. A hot, wet paste wrapped in cloth and applied to the skin.

prostate. A gland surrounding a part of the urethra and neck of the bladder in men. When this gland enlarges, it can result in difficulty in urinating.

prostrate. Lying flat on the ground.

pulp. The soft, inner portion of a fruit.

purgative. Cleans out the intestines or bowels. Some may be administered orally, others rectally.

raceme. A type of spiked inflorescence in which stalked florets grow out of a central stem.

resin. An often sticky plant substance that may ooze slowly or flow freely from a plant that is cut into or broken. Some forms of resin are soluble in oils, others in alcohol; none are soluble in water (unlike gums). Resins dry to a substance that is hard, and may be opaque or translucent. Examples of resin-based products include amber, incense, lacquers, varnishes, turpentine, and sealants and caulkings for such things as boats and wood products. Though chemically and structurally different from latex, the two may be similar in appearance (for example, milky). Resin is a component of all latexes, though not vice-versa. *See also* latex.

rheumatism. A non-specific term which is used to describe muscles or joints that are suffering from inflammation and/or pain.

rhizome. An underground stem that usually grows horizontally and sends out roots and shoots.

ringworm. A superficial fungal infection which causes an itching, scaly condition affecting various parts of the body, such as skin or nails. This condition is caused by one of three genera of fungi (*Microsporum, Trichophyton,* or *Epidermophyton*). Ringworm conditions are usually called *tinea* (Latin for "worm") in combination with another word describing the affected body part; for example, *Tinea pedis* is ringworm of the foot, otherwise known as athlete's foot.

rosette. A cluster of leaves that arises from the base of a plant and forms a circular pattern around the base.

scales. Small leaves, often colorless or pale, often found on stems.

sedative. A treatment which calms or quiets the patient.

segment (of leaf). Each leaflet in a compound leaf.

septic. Having disease-causing bacteria in the bloodstream.

serrate; serrated (leaf). Having small, sharply pointed teeth on the margins.

sheath (of leaf). Basal portion of leaf that wraps around the stem.

sorus (singular); sori (plural). Spore case or cluster of spores found on fern fronds; each sorus may contain thousands of spores. Sori form distinctive markings or patterns that are useful for species identification. *See also* spore.

spadix. An inflorescence of tightly clustered florets growing in a vertical spike that is usually enclosed by a bract (modified leaf) known as a **spathe**.

spasm. A sudden contraction of the muscles.

spasmolytic activity. Ability to stop or slow spasms. *See also* spasm.

spike. An inflorescence in which the flowers appear to grow directly out of a vertically elongated central stem. A **compound spike** is multi-branched.

spine. A leaf that has been modified to become a sharp outgrowth along a stem.

spore. The reproductive part in non-flowering plants such as ferns. Spores are disseminated by wind and water; male and female parts of a spore fuse to become the seed of the next plant. *See also* sorus.

stamen. The male reproductive part of a flower, consisting of the pollen-producing anther which sits atop a stalk (filament).

staminate (flower). Having only the male reproductive parts (stamens).

stipule. An outgrowth at the base of a leaf, usually occurring in pairs.

stomatitis. Mouth inflammation; typical symptoms include heat, pain, and an increased tendency to salivate, among others.

succulent. Juicy; a plant having fleshy stems or leaves which store water.

terminal. Occurring at the end of a branch or stem.

terrestrial. Growing in or out of the ground.

thorn; thorny. A hard, woody, pointed branch, usually much reduced in size.

thrush. A fungal disease of the mouth occurring most often in young children and patients with AIDS. The most common symptoms are the appearance of white patches and ulcerations on the tongue and gums.

tonic. A stimulant or energizer. In local terms, this is often used to "strengthen" blood, muscles, or the entire system.

toothed (leaf). Having a sharply pointed pattern along its margin.

toxic; toxicity; toxin. Poisonous; level of poison; poison.

tristesa. Local Spanish word for sadness and grief.

tuber. Portion of a stem that grows underground and swells to store food reserves for future plant growth.

ulcer. Open wound or sore on skin or mucous membrane. Causes may vary.

unisexual (flowers). Having either male or female reproductive parts, but not both.

varicosity. A vein that is "dilated" and "enlarged." This condition is most common in the lower legs.

vasoconstrictor activity. Ability to constrict blood vessels. *See also* constrict.

vasodilator activity. Ability to dilate blood vessels. *See also* dilate.

veno-occlusive disease of the liver. An obstruction of the veins leading from the liver.

vine. A plant having a flexible stem that cannot stand on its own. Vines commonly attach themselves to other plants or structures that enable them to climb toward sunlight. Although many vines in the tropics have woody stems, they still require the support of other plants.

whorls. The arrangement of the parts of a plant in a concentric pattern with all parts arising from the same point on a stalk. In a complete flower, for example, the whorls consist of (from outermost to innermost) the sepals, petals, stamens, and pistil(s). The term is also applied to other plant parts (for example, leaves, branches, inner rings of tree trunk) that exhibit a similar concentric pattern.

Yucatec. *See* Maya.

References

Bold, H.C., C.J. Alexopoulous, and T. Delevoryas. 1987. *Morphology of Plants and Fungi.* New York, New York: Harper & Row.

GLOSSARY

Core, E.L. and N.P. Ammons. 1958. *Woody Plants in Winter.* Pacific Grove, California: The Boxwood Press.

Heywood, V.H., ed. 1978. *Flowering Plants of the World.* New York, New York: Mayflower Books, Inc.

Newcomb, L. 1977. *Newcomb's Wildflower Guide.* Boston, Massachusetts and Toronto, Canada: Little, Brown and Company.

Peterson, R.T. and M. McKenny. 1968. *A Fieldguide to Wildflowers: Northeastern and North-central North America.* Boston, Massachusetts: Houghton Mifflin Company.

Raven, P.H., R.F. Evert, and S.E. Eichhorn. 1986. *Biology of Plants.* 4th edition. New York, New York: Worth Publishers, Inc.

Smith, C. in collaboration with M. Bermejo Marcos and E. Chang-Rodriguez. 1971. *Collins Spanish-English/English-Spanish Dictionary.* London, England and Glasgow, Scotland: William Collins Sons & Company, Ltd.

Stedman, T.L. 1990. *Stedman's Medical Dictionary.* 25th edition; illustrated. Baltimore, Maryland: Williams & Wilkins.

Thomas, C.L., ed. 1987. *Taber's Cyclopedic Medical Dictionary.* 15th edition; illustrated. Philadelphia, Pennsylvania: F.A. Davis Company.

Webster, N. 1983. *Webster's New Universal Unabridged Dictionary.* Deluxe 2nd edition. Revised by J.L. McKechnie and publisher's editorial staff. New York, New York: New World Dictionaries/Simon and Schuster.

DESCRIPTIONS AND ILLUSTRATIONS

OF PLANTS

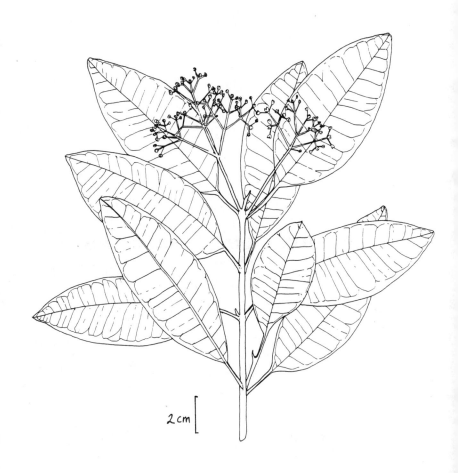

2 cm

Pimenta dioica (L.) Merrill

ALLSPICE

Pimenta, Pimenta Gorda (S)
Naba-cuc (M)

Scientific Name: *Pimenta dioica* (L.) Merrill

Plant Family: Myrtaceae

Description: Tree growing to 20 m tall; stem ca. 30 cm in diameter with light brown bark that peels off in thin strips or larger sheets; leaves leathery, 9-20 cm long x 3-9 cm wide, fragrant; inflorescence a panicle 6-12 cm long, with numerous white flowers ca. 5 mm long; fruits rounded, 6-8 mm in diameter.

Habitat: Forests, backyards.

Traditional Uses: Both the berries and leaves are used medicinally as a pleasant, warming tea for *digestive upsets, gas,* and *infant colic.* Crushed berries boiled down to a paste and spread on a piece of cotton make an excellent plaster for *rheumatic aches and pains.* Those suffering from *exhaustion* or feeling *low in energy* will benefit by bathing with water in which allspice leaves have been boiled. To relieve *menstrual cramps,* take a sitz bath in same. *Chicleros* and lumber workers make a paste of the fresh, crushed allspice berries added to animal fat to apply to *foot fungus.*

The berries are used as a spice for meat stews, hot cereals and liquored drinks, and are collected from wild trees in the forest to be sold for the international spice trade.

Research Results: This plant has been shown to have biological activity as an antifungal. *In vitro* activity against *Lentinus lepideus, Lenzites trabea,* and *Polyporus versicolor* was shown using the essential oil (Maruzzella et al. 1960).

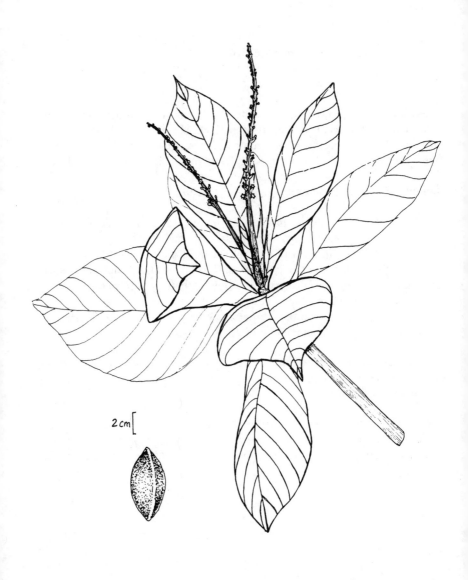

2 cm

Terminalia catappa L.

ALMOND

Almendro (S)
Hammon (C)

Scientific Name: *Terminalia catappa* L.

Plant Family: Combretaceae

Description: A tree growing to 25 m tall, with a stout trunk to 1 m in diameter; branches formed in conspicuous, spreading whorls; leaves 10-30 cm long; flowers in spikes 5-15 cm long; fruits white, shaped like almonds, brown when ripe, 4-7 cm long; seeds 3-4 cm long.

Habitat: Cultivated in yards, orchards, and in public parks and plazas; found also along the sea.

Traditional Uses: Leaves are boiled to make a tea for *high blood pressure* and *heart trouble* -- boil 3 leaves in 3 cups of water for 10 minutes; drink 1 cup every other day, before breakfast. Dosage should not exceed 3 cups weekly as more is said to weaken sex drive.

Research Results: Most of the pharmacological tests on this plant showed no activity. Antibacterial activity was shown using an 80% ethanol extract of dried aerial parts at a concentration of 100 mcg/ml in *Salmonella paratyphi* A *in vitro* (Aynehchi et al. 1982). Analgesic activity was shown in rats using a methanol extract of dried leaf and stem (Esposito-Avella et al. 1985). The plant is known to contain benzenoids, coumarins (Griffiths 1959), lipids (Upadhya et al. 1974), saponins, and tannins (Aynehchi et al. 1985).

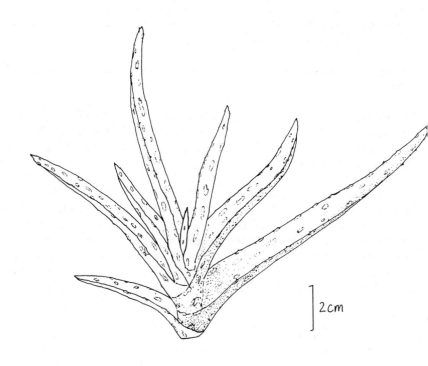

] 2cm

Aloe vera L.

ALOE VERA

Sink-am-Bible (C)

Scientific Name: *Aloe vera* L.

Plant Family: Liliaceae

Description: Small fleshy herb to 60 cm high; leaves narrow, pale green, with small spines along their margins; inflorescence a spike to 1 m tall, with yellow flowers on terminal portion.

Habitat: Cultivated in gardens.

Traditional Uses: Since Biblical times, this has been one of nature's most useful plants. Aloe vera juice is a *purgative* for persons of sedentary habit and weak constitution. For this purpose, mash and soak 1 leaf, about 15 cm in length, in a cup of water for 20 minutes; strain and drink. This will also serve as a *tonic* for the liver, pancreas, kidneys, and stomach. Externally, Aloe vera juice is an excellent remedy for *burns, sunburns, rashes, stubborn ulcers, bed sores, diaper rash, boils, fungus,* and to reduce *scarring.* Apply the juice liberally to the affected area. Note that Aloe vera juice may be harmful when taken internally in excessive amounts.

To remove deeply embedded thorns, stones or fish scales, slice a piece of Aloe vera leaf in half; apply over area and secure with a band or cloth. Leave this dressing on and change once daily -- this will draw out the object in 3-5 days.

Research Results: Aloe vera juice and its extracts have been found effective for a variety of conditions. These include wound healing acceleration in humans (Cobble 1975; Loveman 1937; Barnes 1947); antiviral activities for *herpes simplex* 1 and 2 (Sydiskia and Owen 1987); treatment of hot water burns (Crewe 1939); anti-inflammatory activity in mice (Davis et al. 1991); anesthetic activity for treatment of insect stings in humans (Coutts 1979); and antiulcer activity in rats (Galal et al. 1975). An alcohol extract of *Aloe vera* in drinking water was found to be toxic in mice at a dose of 100 mg/kg for 3 months (Shah et al. 1989). This suggests that caution is warranted for internal, long-term use.

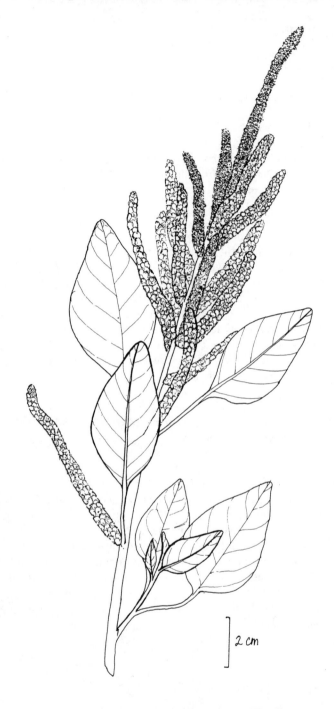

］2 cm

Amaranthus dubius Mart. ex Thell.

AMARANTH

Pig Weed (E)
Quelite (S)
Calaloo (C)

Scientific Name: *Amaranthus dubius* Mart. ex Thell.

Plant Family: Amaranthaceae

Description: Herbaceous plant to 2 m with many branches; leaves dark green, deeply veined; flowers green, borne on drooping spikes at tips of branches; seeds black, shiny, round, ca. 1 mm in diameter.

Habitat: Clearings, yards, roadsides.

Traditional Uses: Leaves and seeds were a food source for the Aztecs and Mayas. Leaves and tender stems are boiled in water and prepared much like spinach. This food is an excellent treatment for *anemia, tiredness, constipation*, and *poor nutrition*.

The entire plant is boiled in water to clean *wounds* and *sores*. Leaves are made into juice to be given as a drink for chronic, advanced states of *anemia* -- drink 1 half cup 3 times daily until well.

The Spanish conquerors were horrified to learn that the Aztecs mixed popped amaranth seed with human blood to form into a ceremonial cake as an offering to their gods. For this reason, it was illegal to cultivate amaranth in New Spain for many generations.

Research Results: The seeds of *Amaranthus dubius* contain lipids, triterpenes, and steroids (Fernando and Bean 1985).

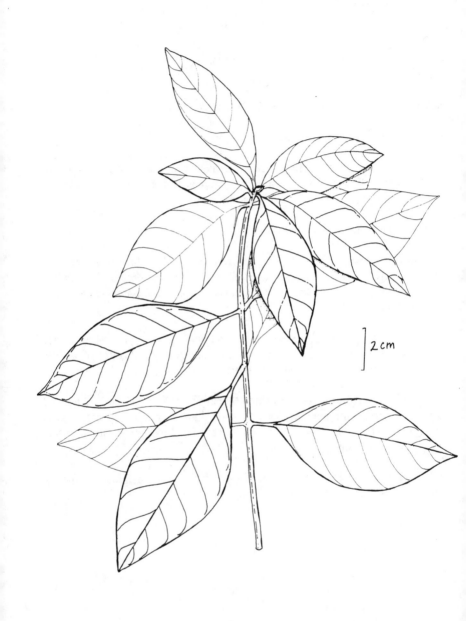

Psychotria acuminata Benth.

ANAL (M)

Ix-Anal (M)

Scientific Name: *Psychotria acuminata* Benth.

Plant Family: Rubiaceae

Description: Woody shrub to 2 m tall; leaves lanceolate, 6-12 cm long and 3-6 cm wide; inflorescence a cluster of yellow flowers ca. 3 mm long; fruits purple, globose, 4-5 mm in diameter.

Habitat: Edge of forests, riversides, disturbed forests.

Traditional Uses: May be used alone or in combination with other leaves to bathe *skin conditions*; to treat those suffering from *rheumatism, nervousness, insomnia, headaches, swellings, bruises*; and for *infantile diseases*. To prepare bath, boil a large double handful of leaves per gallon of water for 10 minutes.

This is the "female" Anal, counterpart to the male Anal (*Psychotria tenuifolia*) discussed on page 71. The concept of male and female plants is common to the Maya pharmacopoeia and there are numerous such "pairs" of plants used in healing.

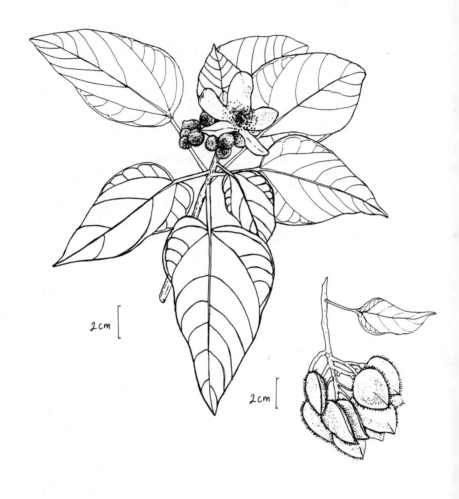

2 cm

2 cm

Bixa orellana L.

12

ANNATTO

Achiote (S)
Ku-xub (M)

Scientific Name: *Bixa orellana* L.

Plant Family: Bixaceae

Description: Woody tree or shrub 2-8 m tall, with a dense rounded shape and short trunk; bark dark brown; leaves green; inflorescences with pink flowers to 5 cm in diameter; capsule ovoid, covered with reddish-brown soft spines; seeds covered with abundant orange-red pulp.

Habitat: Cultivated in yards, orchards, farms.

Traditional Uses: The red pulp surrounding the seeds yields a strong orange-yellow to red dye. The pulp is used as a flavoring and coloring agent.

For *diarrhea* and *dysentery*, crush 3 young leaves in 1 glass of water; strain and drink in 1/2 cup doses. Boil 3 older leaves in 3 cups of water for 10 minutes and drink as a remedy for *vomiting blood*. For *sores, rashes,* and *infected bites*, crush a handful of leaves in water; allow to sit in the sun all day; strain out residue and use as a cool wash. An herbal bath made from the leaves can be used to treat *swellings*. For *stoppage of water*, boil 9 seed pods in 3 cups of water for 10 minutes and drink 1 cup before each meal.

Research Results: An ethyl alcohol extract of dried annatto fruit was shown to have *in vitro* activity against *Escherichia coli* and *Staphylococcus aureus*, and an ethyl alcohol extract of dried leaf was shown to have *in vitro* activity against the same bacteria (George and Pandalai 1949). A water extract of the root was shown to have hypotensive activity in rats and smooth muscle relaxant activity in guinea pigs (Dunham and Allard 1960). A chloroform extract of dried seed was shown to have hypoglycemic activity in dogs (Morrison and West 1985). Annatto leaves contain flavonoids (Harborne 1975) and the seeds contain carotenoids (Tirimanna 1981).

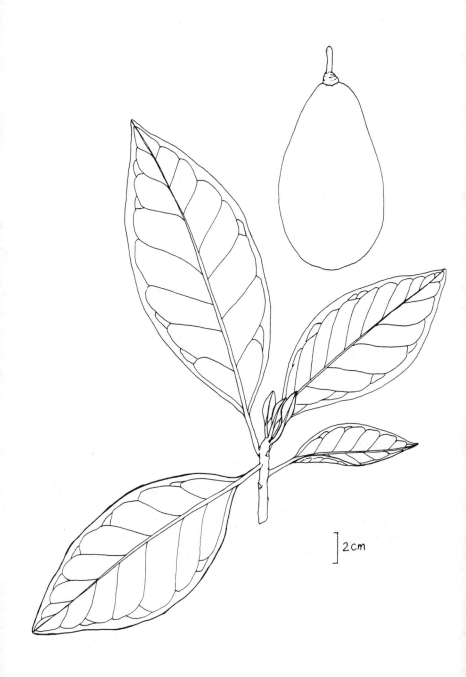

]2cm

Persea americana Mill.

AVOCADO

Avocado Pear (E)
Aguacate (S)

Scientific Name: *Persea americana* Mill.

Plant Family: Lauraceae

Description: Medium to large tree growing to 30 m tall; leaves 10-30 cm long, glabrous; flowers greenish, 5-7 mm long, growing in panicles 6-20 cm long, mostly near the tips of the branches; fruits variable in size, shape (round to pear-shaped), skin color, texture, taste, and flesh color (greenish to brownish).

Habitat: Cultivated, escaped and possibly wild.

Traditional Uses: For *colds, high blood pressure, coughs, fever, diarrhea,* or *painful menses* -- boil 3 leaves in 3 cups of water for 10 minutes and drink 3 cups daily before meals; this is a cooling refrigerant remedy. Make a poultice of the mashed leaves for *headaches, rheumatism,* or *sprains.* Grind or mash the seed; boil in 2 cups water for 10 minutes and drink 1 cup hot 2 times daily for *empacho* (Spanish word for intestinal obstructions).

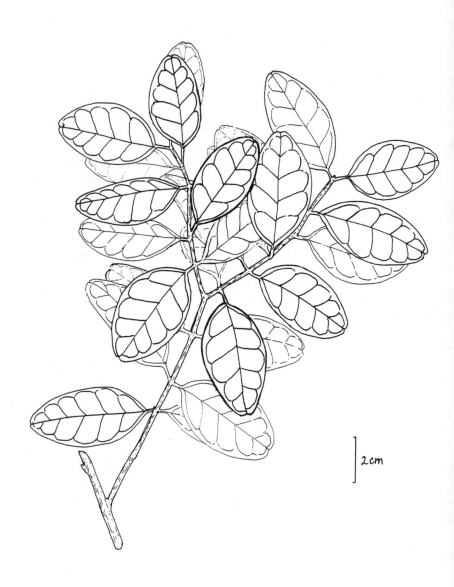

Krugiodendron ferreum (Vahl) Urban.

AX MASTER

Exmasta Bark (E)
Quebracho (S)

Scientific Name: *Krugiodendron ferreum* (Vahl) Urban.

Plant Family: Rhamnaceae

Description: A tree growing to 10 m tall, with a thick trunk to 50 cm in diameter; also found growing as a shrub; leaves 2-7 cm long; flowers yellow-green, 4 mm wide; fruit a black, ovoid or globose drupe, 5-8 mm long.

Habitat: Forests.

Traditional Uses: In our work, we have heard little about the uses of ax master. It appears to be considered a *blood tonic*, similar to provision bark (*Pachira aquatica*). It is available in the Belize City market, and Barbara Fernandez, in her book *Medicine Woman: The Herbal Tradition of Belize* (1990), notes that it is used in mixtures as a tea for *anemia, pleurisy, emphysema*, and *malaria*.

According to Standley and Steyermark (1949), the wood is durable and heavy, with a specific gravity of ca. 1.3.

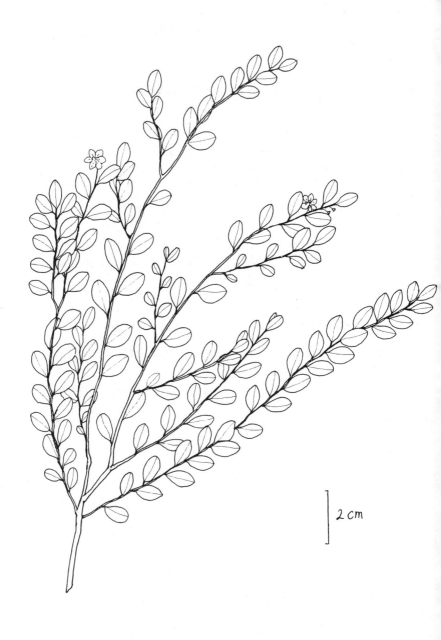

]2 cm

Phyllanthus liebmannianus Muell. Arg.

BABY'S TEARS

Chin-chin-pol-ojo (M)

Scientific Name: *Phyllanthus liebmannianus* Muell. Arg.

Plant Family: Euphorbiaceae

Description: Delicate herb to 50 cm; leaves small, oval-shaped; flowers greenish, hanging from undersides of leaves. Flowering is continuous.

Habitat: Clearings, edge of forests, old fields.

Traditional Uses: Boil an entire plant in 3 cups water for 2 minutes; strain and drink for *stomatitis, internal infections, kidney stones,* and *stoppage of urine.* Use same preparation to *bathe infants* who are ill.

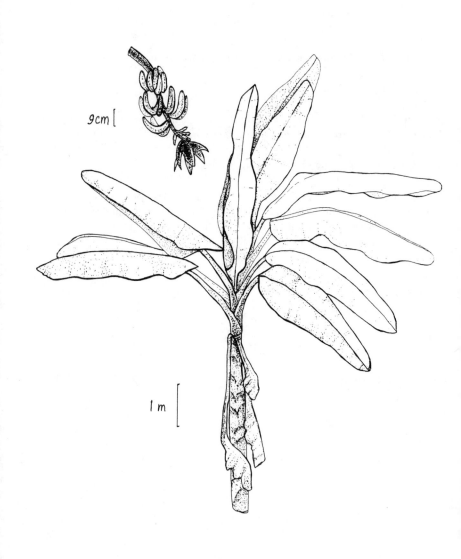

9cm

1 m

Musa acuminata Colla

BANANA

Guineo (S)
Box Haaz (M)

Scientific Name: *Musa acuminata* Colla

Plant Family: Musaceae

Description: Large herb with thick roots, growing to 4 m or more in height; stem fleshy and composed of inrolled leaf sheaths; leaves arranged in a spiral to 1-2 m long; inflorescence a compound spike with unisexual flowers; fruit a fleshy, elongate berry, usually without seeds and deep yellow when ripe.

Habitat: Cultivated on farms, orchards, and yards.

Traditional Uses: An excellent, easily digested tonic food often used as first choice for infants and invalids. Helpful in cases of *gastritis* and *ulcers* when eaten alone. The fresh juice of the stem is rich in potassium and is a powerful *diuretic*; it is also useful for *blisters*, *burns*, and *abscesses*. The root or solid white corm below the ground is used by midwives to staunch excessive *bleeding* in childbirth -- wash root well; grate and squeeze through a porous cloth to obtain liquid; give only 1 tablespoon by mouth every 5 minutes, not to exceed 3 doses. The young, green leaves make an excellent wrap and plaster for *burns* and *blisters*. For *diarrhea*, eat only well-ripened bananas for 24 hours.

Green bananas may be boiled in their skins until tender. Remove skins and mash; then form into cakes and cook as for *tortillas* or pancakes.

Research Results: A great deal of research has been carried out on this popular fruit. Weak anti-tuberculosis activity was demonstrated in an agar plate culture of *Mycobacterium tuberculosis*, using fruit juice (Fitzpatrick 1954). Antiulcer activity in rats was shown using a dose of 5 gm/animal of fruit in the ration, both before and after aspirin treatment (Best et al. 1984). *In vitro* antibacterial activity was shown against *Bacillus cereus*, *Bacillus coagulans*, *Bacillus stereothermophilus*, and *Clostridium sporogenes* using a water extract of concentrated banana puree (Richter and Vore 1989).

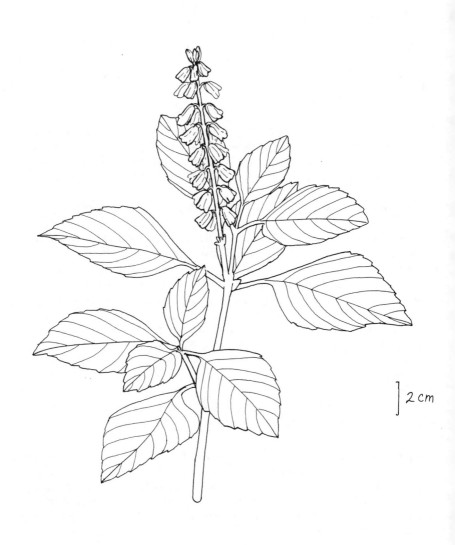

]2 cm

Ocimum basilicum L.

BASIL

Alboharcar (S)
Ca-cal-tun (M)
Barsley, Balsley (C)

Scientific Name: *Ocimum basilicum* L.

Plant Family: Lamiaceae

Description: Herb growing to 50 cm; stem usually square (especially when young), bearing many branches; leaves highly aromatic, each 2-4 cm long; flowers green, borne on spikes that turn brown when seed matures.

Habitat: Gardens, backyards, roadsides and fields.

Traditional Uses: To promote delayed *menstruation*, ease pain of *difficult menstruation*, and to facilitate *childbirth* -- boil one entire plant in 3 cups water for 2 minutes; steep 20 minutes and give to drink warm. Boil entire plant to use as *vaginal steam bath* after delivery. Boil a small handful of fresh leaves in 2 cups water for 2 minutes and steep for 20 minutes; drink for *stomachache, intestinal parasites*, and to *induce perspiration in feverish conditions*. Tiny dried seeds are placed in eye and left in overnight to rid eyes of *phlegm* and as a minor aid to discourge the formation of *cataracts*. Leaf is dried and powdered to be applied to *sores*, especially those containing *worms* or *larvae*. Drop leaf juice into ear for *earache*.

Fresh or dried leaves may be added to soup, meat sauces, tomato dishes, and salads.

Research Results: The essential oil from this species displayed *in vitro* antibacterial activity against *Bacillus subtilis, Escherichia coli, Pseudomonas aeruginosa*, and *Staphylococcus aureus*, and antiyeast activity against *Candida albicans* (Janssen et al. 1986). Insecticidal activity against *Colex quinquefasciatus* was obtained using a petroleum ether extract at a concentration of 100 PPM (parts per million) from the dried plant (Kalyanasundaram and Babu 1982). Essential oil showed *in vitro* antifungal activity against *Lonzites trabea, Polyporus versicolor*, and several plant pathogens at an unspecified concentration (Maruzzella et al. 1960). Antiascariasis activity was shown using a water extract of the leaf for earthworms (Jain and Jain 1972).

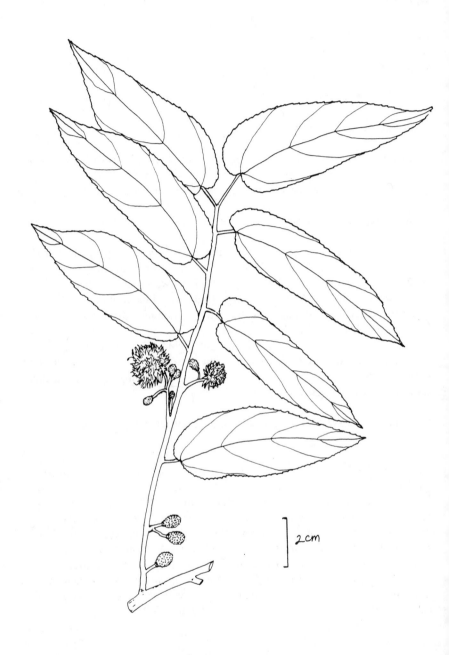

Guazuma ulmifolia Lam.

BAY CEDAR

Pixoy (M)

Scientific Name: *Guazuma ulmifolia* Lam.

Plant Family: Sterculiaceae

Description: Large shrub or tree to 12 m tall; stem to ca. 25 cm in diameter with gray-brown bark; leaves 5-15 cm long with serrated edges; flowers small, greenish-yellow to white, fragrant; fruit woody, globose to broadly oval, 2-4 cm long, black when ripe, covered with rough barbs.

Habitat: Pastures, fields and disturbed areas, forests.

Traditional Uses: For *dysentery* and *diarrhea*, boil a small handful of chopped bark in 3 cups of water for 10 minutes; drink 3 cups daily, 1 before each meal. Drink same decoction for *prostate* problems (add honey), and as an aid to *childbirth* (sip slowly). As a wash for *skin sores, infections*, and *rashes*, boil a large handful of chopped bark in a gallon of water for 10 minutes; allow to cool and bathe affected area 3 times daily; do not dry with towel -- allow to air dry.

Children like to eat these sweet fruits, but are likely to get constipated due to the presence of tannic acid. The fruit is an excellent food for grazing animals. It is also eaten by birds, squirrels, and other forest animals.

Research Results: The leaf is known to contain 0.09-0.14% caffeine (Freise 1935), and the bark to contain tannins (Domínguez S. and Alcorn 1985). An ethanol (95%) extract of dried leaf showed *in vitro* cytotoxic activity against 9KB cancer cells, giving a 97.3% inhibition of cell growth (Nascimento et al. 1990). *In vitro* antibacterial activity was exhibited by a dried leaf tincture against *Bacillus subtilis* at a concentration of 0.1 ml per disc (an extract of 10 gm plant material in 100 ml of ethanol) (Cáceres et al. 1987). The same study noted *in vitro* activity against *Escherichia coli* from a similar tincture used at a concentration of 30 mcl per disc. Uterine stimulant effect in a rat was shown using a water extract of stem bark; the concentration was not noted (Barros et al. 1970).

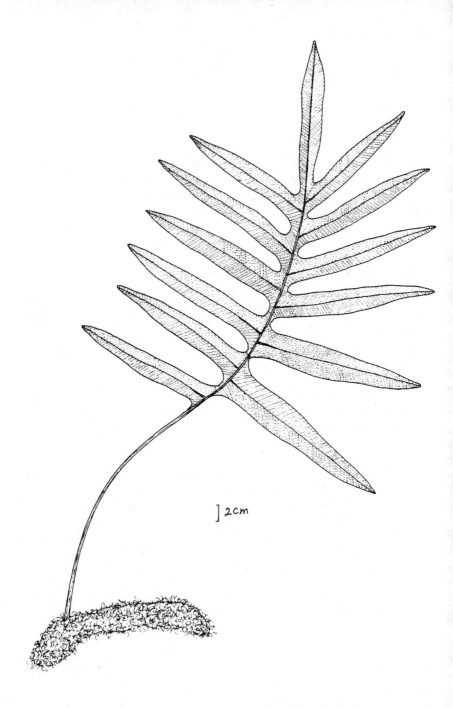

] 2cm

Phlebodium decumanum (Willd.) J. Smith

BEAR PAW FERN

Callawalla, Tallawalla, Canawana (S)

Scientific Name: *Phlebodium decumanum* (Willd.) J. Smith

Plant Family: Polypodiaceae

Description: Epiphytic plants, or occasionally terrestrial, with thick (2 cm) rhizomes covered with orange scales; leaves large, to 40-160 cm long, on 12-55 cm long petioles, each leaf with 4-10 pairs of segments; sori (spore capsules) brown and round, with several occuring between mid-vein and leaf margin.

Habitat: Found growing as a parasite in cohune (*Orbignya cohune*) palms.

Traditional Uses: An excellent remedy for *stomach ulcers, pain, gastritis,* and *chronic indigestion* -- boil a piece of root 8 cm long in 2 cups water for 10 minutes; drink 1/2 cup 4 times daily for 6 weeks. The plant is known throughout Belize for the treatment of "cancer," a word describing a type of open sore. Local herbalists recommend drinking the same decoction for beginning stages of *cancer, pain of latter stages,* and *high blood pressure.*

Research Results: It appears that little pharmacological work has been carried out with this species, despite its widespread use. It is known to contain carotenoids (Czeczuga 1985), flavonoids (Gómez and Wallace 1986), and steroids (Ganguly and Sircar 1974).

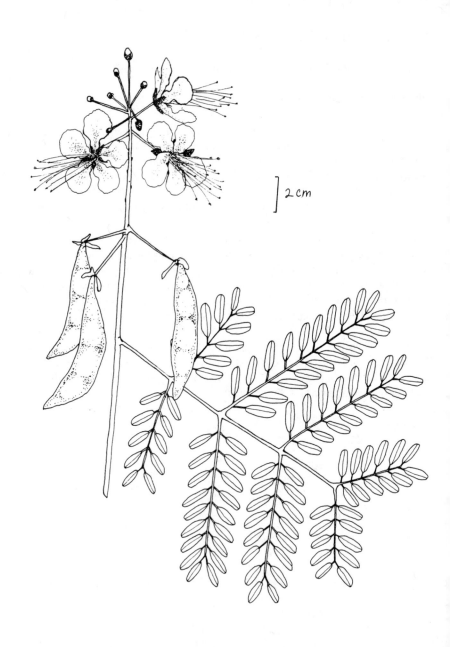

Caesalpinia pulcherrima (L.) Sw.

BIRD OF PARADISE FLOWER

Flambeau Flower (E)
Irritación, Flor de la Virgen (S)
Chink-in, Can-zink-in (M)

Scientific Name: *Caesalpinia pulcherrima* (L.) Sw.

Plant Family: Caesalpiniaceae

Description: Shrub or small tree to 5 m tall; branches brittle; leaves large with 3-9 pairs of pinnae, 6-12 pairs of leaflets; flowers red or bright yellow, to 5 cm across; fruit a pod, 12 cm long x 1.5-2 cm wide.

Habitat: Cleared fields, backyards, fences.

Traditional Uses: For *"irritación,"* an infantile disease characterized by *fever, swollen belly, cold hands and feet, perspiration*, and *diarrhea* -- squeeze a large double handful of leaves in 1 gallon of hot water and allow to soak in sun all day; bathe infant with this warm sun tea for 3 nights and give 1/4 cup to drink after each bath. For both children and adults suffering from *"tristesa"* -- sadness and grief -- bathe in this mixture.

The flowers yield a good quality honey. It is said that if you "lash" small children who show bad tempers with a switch from this plant and throw the switch over the house roof at noon, they will stop misbehaving.

The green seeds found in the pods are edible.

Research Results: A methyl alcohol extract of the dried bark of Bird of Paradise flower was shown to have *in vitro* activity against *Staphylococcus aureus* (Khan et al. 1980), and a water extract of the fresh leaves was shown to have strong *in vitro* antifungal activity against *Ustilago maydis* and *Ustilago nuda*, both plant pathogens (Singh and Pathak 1984). A methanol extract of dried root bark was shown to have *in vitro* activity against *Staphylococcus aureus* and *Escherichia coli* (Khan et al. 1980). Note that an ethanol-chloroform extract of fresh seed pods was shown to have tumor promoting effect (94% enhancement of sarcoma HS1 tumor) in mice (Caldwell and Brewer 1983).

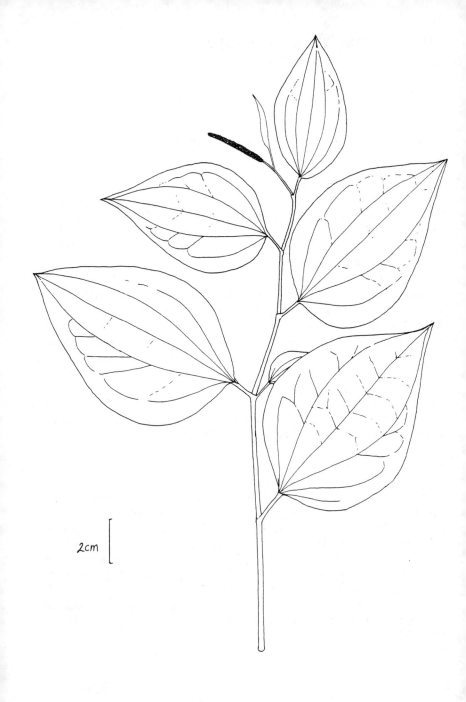

2cm

Piper amalago L.

30

BUTTONWOOD

Spanish Elder (E)
Cordonsillo (S)

Scientific Name: *Piper amalago* L.

Plant Family: Piperaceae

Description: A slender, much branched shrub to 1.5-3 m tall; branches shiny; leaves 7-14 cm long x 3.5-7 cm wide; flowers in greenish or white spikes each 3-7 cm long and 2.5 mm thick.

Habitat: Forests, old fields, roadsides, and backyards.

Traditional Uses: All species of *Piper* may be used for herbal baths. In cases of *aches, pains, rheumatism, swellings, skin conditions, fatigue*, and *sleeplessness*, boil a large double handful of freshly picked leaves in 2 gallons of water; allow to cool to very warm and bathe by soaking in tub or pouring over body using a bowl as a scooper. Roots of all varieties of this plant family are used to alleviate *toothaches* -- dig up a portion of root; mash into a poultice and apply over gum area and retain. As first aid for *snakebite*, boil a piece of root equal to length of victim's forearm in 3 cups of water for 10 minutes, and give to victim to drink while being transported to hospital or snake doctor. Also for snakebite, boil 9 mature leaves in 3 cups of water for 5 minutes and drink 1 cup before meals. Mash leaves and drink cold for *headache, constipation*, and as a *sedative*. For women with *menstrual cramps* or *delayed menses*, soak 20 minutes in a sitz bath before bedtime for 3 consecutive nights.

Research Results: Dried bark of this species, in a methanol extract, showed molluscicidal activity against snails at 50 PPM (Domínguez S. and Alcorn 1985). Spasmolytic activity in guinea pig ileum was reported using a water extract of fresh leaf and stem at .033 ml/l (Feng et al. 1962). This same reference reported that an ethanol extract (95%) showed spasmolytic activity in guinea pigs, and vasoconstrictor activity from a similar extract in rats. Hypertensive activity in dogs was shown in water and 95% ethanol leaf and stem extracts at a dose of 0.1 ml/kg (ibid.). The species is known to contain triterpenes, steroids (Domínguez S. and Alcorn 1985), proteids, alkaloids (Durand et al. 1962), and sesquiterpenes (Achenbach et al. 1984.)

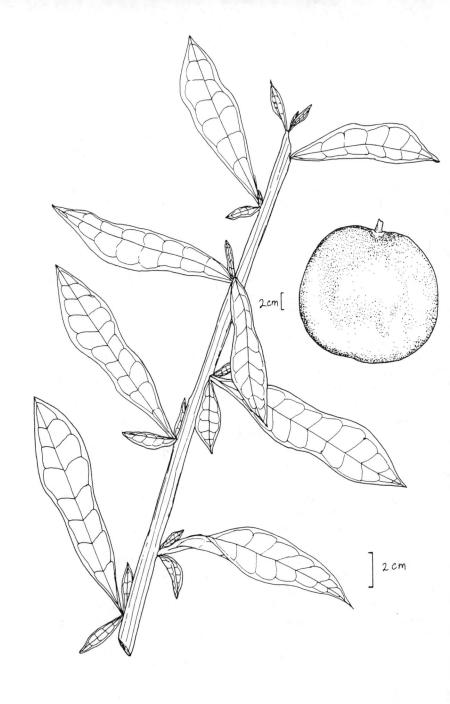

2cm[

] 2 cm

Crescentia cujete L.

CALABASH TREE

Scientific Name: *Crescentia cujete* L.

Plant Family: Bignoniaceae

Description: Tree growing to 5 m tall; leaves few, entire, green; fruits shiny green, globe-shaped, 25 cm in diameter with white, stringy, seedy pith inside.

Habitat: Scrub forests, roadsides, yards.

Traditional Uses: Boil inner, stringy pith of 1 mature fruit with 2 cups sugar and two quarts water for 30 minutes; strain and take by spoonful 6 times daily for *asthma, bronchitis, coughs*, and *lung congestion*. When fruits are not available, boil a handful of leaves in 3 cups of water and 1/2 cup sugar for 30 minutes; take as above.

When pith is removed, dried fruit makes fine bowls and containers.

Research Results: Uses elsewhere include the seed as an abortive (González and Silva 1987), and the fruit pulp to force menses, birth, and afterbirth (Ayensu 1978). Consequently, it is best not to consume this plant while pregnant. Dried bark shows *in vitro* antibacterial activity against *Bacillus subtilis, Pseudomonas aeruginosa, Staphylococcos aureus,* and *Escherichia coli* (Verpoorte and Dihal 1987). The TRAMIL 4 workshop recommended against the internal use of the pulp based on its toxicity (Robineau 1991). Caution is, therefore, advised.

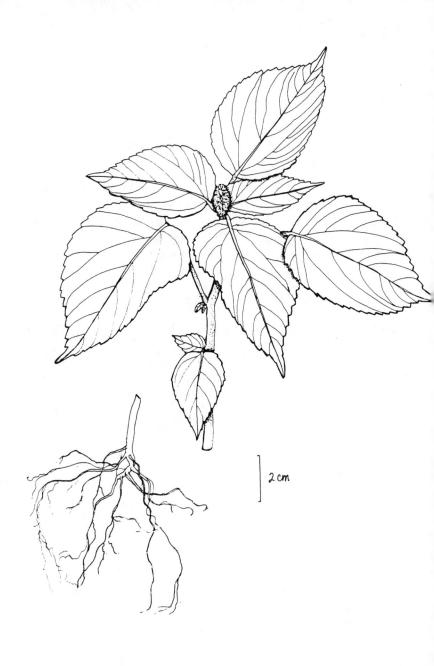

Acalypha arvensis Poepp. & Endl.

CANCER HERB

Hierba del Cancer (S)

Scientific Name: *Acalypha arvensis* Poepp. & Endl.

Plant Family: Euphorbiaceae

Description: Herb to 50 cm tall, often growing in groups of several plants; flowers green, in short spikes.

Habitat: Old fields, yards, other disturbed sites.

Traditional Uses: Excellent remedy to wash *skin conditions* of the worst kind such as *chronic rashes, blisters, peeling skin, deep sores, ulcers, fungus, ringworm, inflammation, itching and burning of labia in women* -- boil one entire plant in one quart water for 10 minutes; strain and wash area with very hot water 3 times daily. Leaves may be dried and toasted and passed through a screen to make a powder to sprinkle on *sores, skin infections,* or *boils*. For *stomach complaints* or *urinary infections*, boil one entire plant in 3 cups water for 5 minutes; drink 3 cups of warm decoction 3 times a day (1 cup before each meal). As mentioned under Bear Paw Fern (p. 25), the local use of the word "cancer" refers to a type of open sore.

Research Results: A dried leaf tincture was shown to have *in vitro* activity against *Staphylococcus aureus*; it was shown to be inactive against *Escherichia coli, Pseudomonas aeruginosa*, and *Candida albicans* (Cáceres et al. 1987). In an *in vitro* human colon cancer screen, extracts of dried leaf and twigs were found to be inactive (Chapuis et al. 1988).

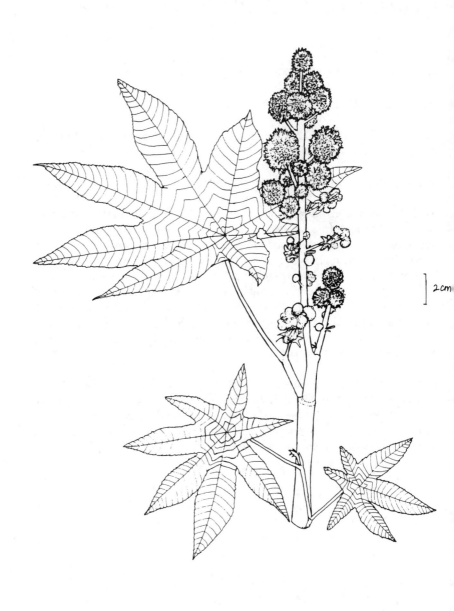

2cm

Ricinus communis L.

CASTOR BEAN PLANT

Oil Nut (E)
Ricino, Higuera (S)
Xcoch (M)

Scientific Name: *Ricinus communis* L.

Plant Family: Euphorbiaceae

Description: Erect shrub or small tree to 6 m tall; trunk to 4 cm in diameter; leaves deeply lobed, 10-60 cm across; flowers in a spike, purple brown in color; fruits brown, 1.5-2.5 cm long; seeds black or mottled brown-creme, each 10-17 mm long.

Habitat: Old fields, roadsides, edge of forest, gardens.

Traditional Uses: Seeds and leaves have been used since ancient times as a *purgative* and *emollient*. Boil 1/2 of a leaf plus 5 dried seeds in 2 cups water for 5 minutes and drink warm as a *purgative*. Use 1/2 leaf plus 2 seeds in same manner as a *laxative*. Crush fresh leaves into paste to apply to *cuts, sores,* and *swellings* to improve healing time. For *pain*, heat a large leaf in oil and apply to area as a poultice overnight. For *headaches* and *sinus congestion*, apply small amount of "Vicks" to forehead; wrap with castor leaf; tie with cloth and lie down for 1 hour or use at bedtime. Boil 5 large leaves in 2 gallons water for 10 minutes to bathe children with *measles* (alleviates itching and prevents scarring). Steam from boiled leaves is used as a *vaginal treatment* for female disorders (e.g., *vaginal tract infections* and *post childbirth pains*). For *fevers*, heat leaf in oil; rub over body and wrap up warm overnight.

Research Results: The seeds, and to some extent the foliage, are poisonous, containing the compound ricin (Kingsbury 1964). Ricin is said to have "many of the poisonous characteristics of a bacterial toxin" (p. 194) and pure ricin is one of the most poisonous compounds known. Heat inactivates the ricin (a protein) contained in the seeds (Farnsworth 1993). An ethanol-water (1:1) extract of the leaf showed antiviral activity at a concentration of 50 mcg/ml against *Vaccinia* virus (Dhar et al. 1968). An ethanol (95%) extract of the leaf showed galactagogue effect at a dose of 3.75 ml/person (Gilfillan 1862).

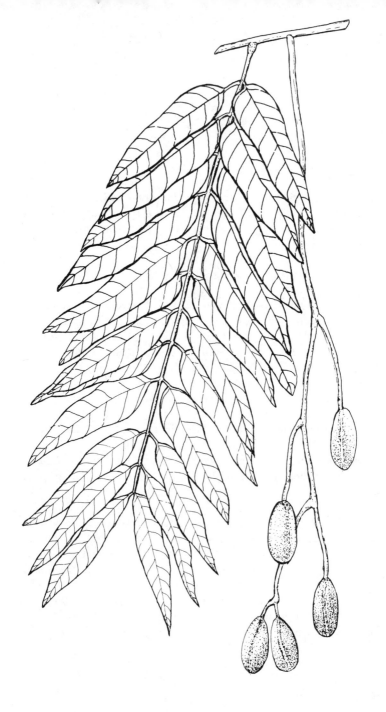

] 2 cm

Cedrela odorata L.

CEDAR

Cedro (S)
Ku-che (M)

Scientific Name: *Cedrela odorata* L.

Plant Family: Meliaceae

Description: A tree to 20-30 m tall, with a stout trunk to 1 m in diameter; wood with strong odor; leaves with 10-30 leaflets, each 7-13 cm long and 2.5-4.5 cm wide; flowers small, white, with glabrous filaments; fruit a capsule ca. 4 cm long; seeds with a 12-20 mm long wing.

Habitat: Forests, clearings.

Traditional Uses: Soak handful of grated bark in 3 cups of water for 6 hours; drink in sips all day for *bruises, falls, postoperative states, internal injuries, abdominal pain,* and to clear lungs of *mucus.* The bark is bitter and used as a tonic (Standley and Steyermark 1946).

This tree is widely harvested for use as timber, and has been appreciated since ancient times for its durability. It is resistant to insect attacks, presumably due to the presence of a volatile oil in the wood (ibid.).

Research Results: Relative to the vast distribution and importance of this species as a timber and in medicine, little research has been carried out on it. Dried bark has shown molluscicidal activity and germination inhibition on corn and beans at 50 PPM in a methanol extract (Domínguez S. and Alcorn 1985). The fresh leaf and stem has shown hypotensive activity in dogs (95% ethanol extract, 0.1 ml/kg dose) (Feng et al. 1962). The minimum toxic dose of a fresh leaf ethanol extract in mice was shown to be 1 ml/animal; in a water extract the toxic dose was shown to be 0.1 ml/animal (ibid.). Vasodilator activity in rats was found from a 95% ethanol fresh leaf extract (concentration of 0.33 ml/l) in rats (ibid.).

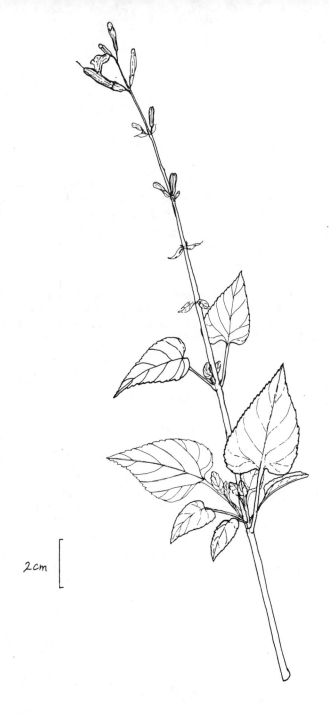

2cm

Salvia coccinea Buc'hoz ex Etling.

40

CHACALPEC (M)

Chac-te-pec (M)

Scientific Name: *Salvia coccinea* Buc'hoz ex Etling.

Plant Family: Lamiaceae

Description: Annual or perennial herb, to 2 m tall; stems slender, branched, usually square (especially when young); leaves 3-6 cm long; flowers 13-20 mm long, red, in thin racemes.

Habitat: Disturbed areas, roadsides.

Traditional Uses: Boil several large plants in 1 gallon of water for 10 minutes; use warm to bathe *varicosities, blood clots,* and *congested blood* ("pasmo" in Spanish).

Research Results: Flavonoids have been identified from the flowers (Tomas-Barberan et al. 1987). The entire plant contains alkanes, steroids, triterpenes (Mukherjee and Ghosh 1978), and diterpenes have been found in the aerial parts (Savona et al. 1982).

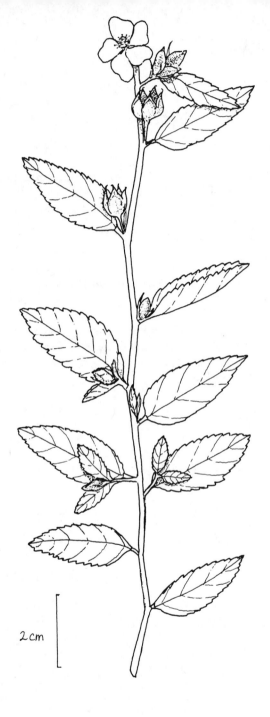

2cm

Sida rhombifolia L.

CHICHIBE (M)

Escoba, Malva (S)

Scientific Name: *Sida rhombifolia* L.

Plant Family: Malvaceae

Description: A low shrub or herb; stems woody, growing to 50-150 cm tall; leaves ca. 1-2 cm long, tinted red, with pointed tips; flowers solitary, yellow, forming in the leaf axils, each ca. 1 cm across, opening at noon.

Habitat: Common in old fields, lots, roadsides.

Traditional Uses: For *burning in urine, stoppage of urine, gonorrhea,* and as an *expectorant* to loosen *dry coughs,* boil about 1 cup fresh leaves in 3 cups of water for 5 minutes; drink 1 cup before each meal. Mash root and apply as poultice to *sprains.*

The common name in Spanish ("escoba") refers to this plant's use as a broom. The fresh, erect stems and leaves are bound to a thin pole and used to sweep out the house and yard.

Research Results: Antibacterial effect was shown *in vitro* on agar plate from an alkaloid fractionation of aerial parts at a concentration of 1 mg/ml in *Escherichia coli, Bacillus subtilis, Bacillus anthracis, Pseudomonas aeruginosa, Staphylococcos aureus,* and *Klebsiella pneumoniae* (Mishra and Chaturvedi 1978). The same study showed *in vitro* antifungal activity of an alkaloid fractionation of aerial parts at a concentration of 1 mg/ml in several plant pathogenic fungi.

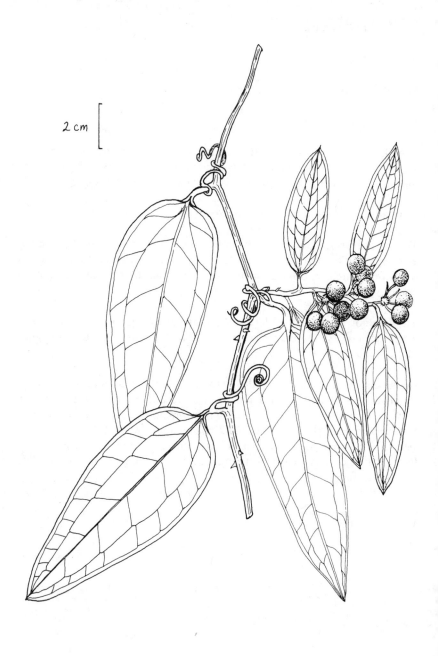

Smilax aff. *lanceolata* L.

CHINA ROOT

Red China Root (E)

Scientific Name: *Smilax* aff. *lanceolata* L.

Plant Family: Smilacaceae

Description: A thorny vine growing up into the forest canopy, with an underground red tuber; leaves lanceolate (heart-shaped in some species), to 9 cm long by 5 cm wide, shiny and smooth; flowers small, greenish; fruit a brown berry, 5-10 mm long.

Habitat: Forests, undisturbed areas.

Traditional Uses: Chop and boil a small handful of roots in 3 cups of water to use as a pleasant tasting *blood tonic* and for *fatigue, anemia, acidity, toxicity, rheumatism,* and *skin conditions.* Drink with milk, cinnamon, and nutmeg to strengthen and proliferate red blood cells.

Research Results: The genus *Smilax* contains some 200 species, widely distributed in temperate and tropical areas around the world. Some species have been tested in pharmacological laboratories and have shown biological activity. No information was found for *Smilax lanceolata.*

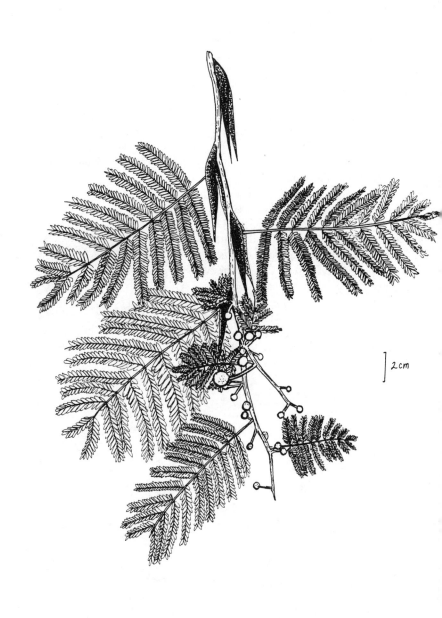

Acacia cornigera (L.) Willd.

COCKSPUR

Subin, Zubin (M)

Scientific Name: *Acacia cornigera* (L.) Willd.

Plant Family: Mimosaceae

Description: Shrub or small tree to 6 m; pinnate leaves with large black spines up to 8 cm long, inhabited by stinging ants; flowers yellow; fruit a dark red pod, 4-5 cm long and 1 cm thick, with pointed tip.

Habitat: Disturbed forests and roadsides.

Traditional Uses: Root and bark are used in *snakebite remedy*. Bushmasters instruct that the snakebite victim should cut a piece of the bark equal to his forearm and chew this, swallowing the juices, and applying the leftover fibers as a poultice to the bite; the victim can then start walking home while chewing on the root and swallowing the juice. The poultice is said to delay reaction time to the toxin, adding 6-8 hours of time to allow victim to get help.

For *male impotency*, boil a 2.5 x 15 cm strip of bark in 3 cups water for 10 minutes and take 1 cup before meals for 7 days. If results are slow, double the strength of the tea for 3 more days. For *infantile catarrh*, catch 9 of the small black ants that inhabit the thorns (they protect the tree from attack from harmful insects); squeeze these into 1/2 cup boiled water; strain and give to infant by teaspoon until consumed. For onset of *asthma attacks, cough*, and *lung congestion*, boil 9 thorns (including their ants) in 3 cups of water for 10 minutes. Said to be useful also for treatment of *poisoning* and *headaches*.

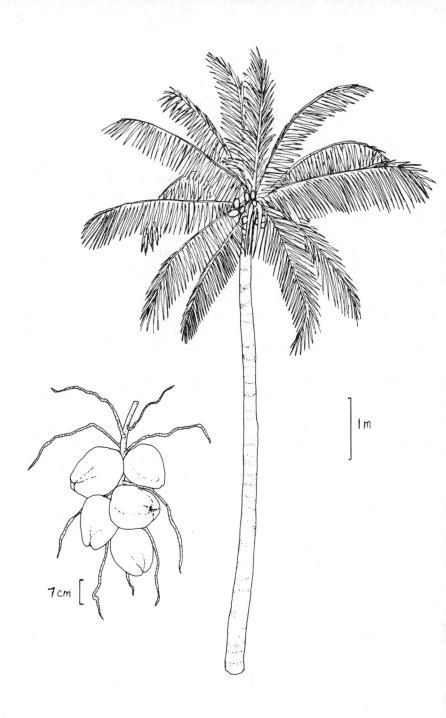

1 m

7 cm

Cocos nucifera L.

COCONUT

Coco (S)

Scientific Name: *Cocos nucifera* L.

Plant Family: Arecaceae

Description: Palm to 20 m in height with a stout trunk to 50 cm in diameter; leaves to 5 m or longer, with regularly spaced pinnae giving a graceful appearance; fruit ovoid, green, containing a large seed to ca. 20 cm long filled with liquid endosperm (if unripe) or a white "meat" (when mature).

Habitat: Seaside, beaches, fields where it is cultivated and escaped.

Traditional Uses: The kernel or endosperm (beneath the hard shell) is the part largely consumed as food. When very young, this kernel is a jelly-like substance, free from fiber and easily digested. Therefore, it can be safely given to children with mashed banana as a *first food*; to those suffering from *indigestion, gastric ulcers, colitis, hepatitis,* and *diarrhea*; and to those in *weakened conditions*. Boil 2 very young fruits while about 3-4 inches in length in 1 cup of water for 10 minutes to relieve *infant diarrhea*; give by spoonful all day. It is a good food for *diabetics* because it contains no fat or starch. Tender coconut flesh is an excellent cosmetic wash to keep the face clean of *pimples* and *prevent wrinkles*. To *eradicate tapeworm*, drink a glassful of coconut milk in the morning, followed by 1 ounce of castor oil a few hours later. Coconut milk is used as a *cooling medicine* mixed with lemon. Tender coconut water (from immature fruit) is a rich source of potassium and other minerals. Its use is recommended in *heart, liver,* and *kidney* disorders; *toxemia of pregnancy*; high *acidity of urine*; and *gonorrhea*. In *kidney failure*, tender coconut water should be given only by a physician. For *dehydration* of adults, children, and infants, tender coconut water mixed with lime juice is an excellent remedy. This water can be mixed with infant formula to prevent curdling of milk in the stomach as well as *vomiting, constipation,* and *indigestion*. Mixed with a tablespoon of honey, it is a good *nerve tonic* and useful for *bronchitis, constipation,* and *piles*.

Research Results: A 95% ethanol extract of dried coconut shell at a concentration of 100 mcg/ml showed *in vitro* activity against *Microsporum audouini, Microsporum canis, Microsporum gypseum, Trichophyton rubrum, Trichophyton tonsurans, Trichophyton violaceum,* and *Epidermophyton floccosum* (Venkataraman et al. 1980). This species is widely used in folk medicine around the world. There appears a paucity of pharmacological testing to verify the efficacy of these uses.

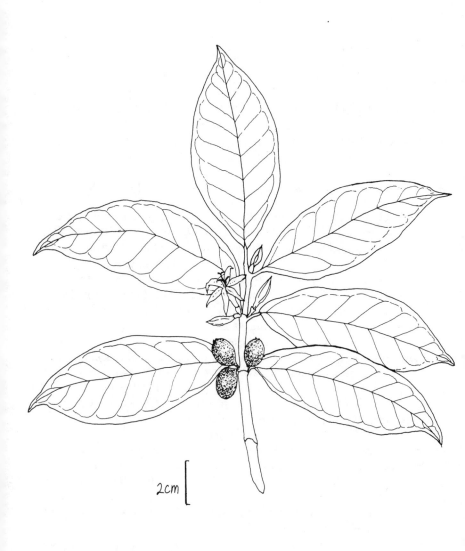

2cm

Coffea arabica L.

COFFEE

Café (S)

Scientific Name: *Coffea arabica* L.

Plant Family: Rubiaceae

Description: Shrub or small tree to 5.5 m tall; leaves dark green, shiny, 7-20 cm long; flowers white, in clusters of 2-9 and very fragrant; fruits ovoid, green turning red, then blue-black, ca. 1 cm long.

Habitat: Cultivated in plantations or in dooryard gardens.

Traditional Uses: As a *stimulant*, boil 3 leaves in 1 cup of water for 10 minutes and drink hot. Also prepared in this way for use as a *diuretic*. Ripe fruit flesh is *edible*. Shells of green, unroasted coffee seeds exude a resin when mashed -- this is placed on a piece of cloth to apply to soles and forehead of infants suffering with *fever*.

Research Results: Chemical analyses of the leaves has shown that they contain allantoic acid, allantoin (Hofmann et al. 1969), caffeine, theobromine (Frischknecht et al. 1986), histidine (Hofman et al. 1969), and the flavonoid quercetin-3-0-alpha-glucoside (González et al. 1975).

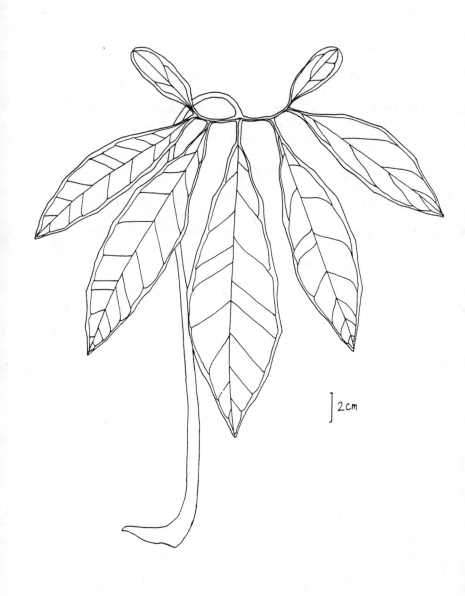

Syngonium podophyllum Schott

52

CONTRA HIERBA (S)

Consuelda, Hinchazón (S)
Hop-ya (M)

Scientific Name: *Syngonium podophyllum* Schott

Plant Family: Araceae

Description: A vine growing to 5 m tall; leaves large, deeply lobed; fruits red; sticky latex exudes from plant when stem or leaf is broken.

Habitat: Parasitic vine growing on trees in forest clearings.

Traditional Uses: Boil 9 leaves in 1 gallon water for 10 minutes -- use warm as a wash for *skin conditions, sores, dry skin, fungus, itching, rashes,* and *bruises.* For *rheumatism, arthritis, pains,* and *swellings,* soak 3 large leaves in 1 quart of alcohol for 7 days in the sun; rub on painful area 3 times daily with cotton.

For *rectal bleeding in dogs,* apply juice of mashed leaves.

Research Results: Plants in this family often contain calcium oxalate crystals which, if ingested, can be quite irritating to internal tissue, and even toxic (Kingsbury 1964). Caution is, therefore, advised.

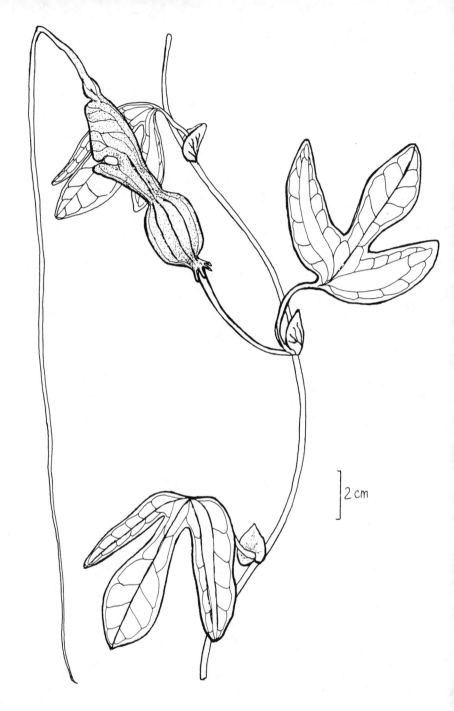

Aristolochia trilobata L.

CONTRIBO (S)

Duck Flower (E)
Flor de Pato (S)

Scientific Name: *Aristolochia trilobata* L.

Plant Family: Aristolochiaceae

Description: Vining plant to 3 m tall; stems slender with dark, rough bark which peels off easily and emits a strong characteristic odor; leaves dark green with three lobes; flower when closed is pale pink and has the shape of a duck; open flower can be up to 20 cm across and is speckled with brown and mauve with a brownish cord-like appendage to 50 cm long; the seed pod is brown and in the shape of a cylindrical basket.

Habitat: Forests, riversides in undisturbed areas.

Traditional Uses: One of the most popular herbal remedies of Belize. Contribo can often be seen soaking in a bottle of rum at saloons as it is taken by the shot for *hangovers, flu, colds, constipation, stomachache, indigestion, flatulence, gastritis, amoebas, colitis, high blood pressure, to clean urinary tract, for "heavy" heartbeat, loss of appetite,* and for scanty or late *menses.* For tea, boil a small handful of chopped vine in 3 cups of water for 10 minutes; strain and drink 1 cup of warm tea before meals as needed. Avoid drinking cold liquids while taking this herb.

For the weak or aged, avoid boiling vine, but rather soak it in water all day and then give 1 cup 3 times daily before meals.

Research Results: Extracts of the stem of contribo were tested for antimalarial activity in animal models and were found to be inactive (Spencer et al. 1947). It is found to be inactive when tested for insecticidal activity for several species of insects (Heal et al. 1950). It appears that very little research has been carried out on this species. Aristolochic acid, found within this genus, is known to be both mutagenic and carcinogenic in animals. Use of this plant on a continuous basis cannot be recommended (Farnsworth 1993).

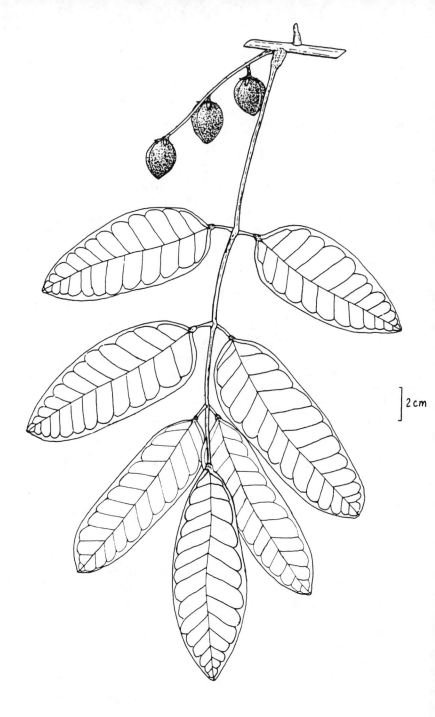

Protium copal (Schlecht. & Cham.) Engler

56

COPAL (S)

Pom (M)

Scientific Name: *Protium copal* (Schlecht. & Cham.) Engler

Plant Family: Burseraceae

Description: A tree growing to 30 m tall, with thick trunk to 50 cm in diameter; leaves large, 10-18 cm long, somewhat leathery; inflorescence a panicle, ca. 12 cm long; fruit 1.5-3 cm long, glabrous.

Habitat: Forests.

Traditional Uses: *Chicleros* who stayed in the bush for months relied on fresh copal resin to treat *painful cavities* -- a piece of resin was stuffed into the cavity and, in a few days, the tooth broke apart and was easily expelled. The bark is scraped, powdered and applied to *wounds, sores,* and *infections.* Cut a piece of bark 2.5 cm x 15 cm; boil in 3 cups of water for 10 minutes and drink 1 cup before meals for *stomach complaints* and *intestinal parasites.*

Copal is one of the sacred trees of the ancient Maya who used the resin for ceremonial incense in prayer and to ward off *witchcraft, evil spirits,* and the *"evil eye."* According to an old Mayan custom, the tree bark is sliced open on a night when the moon is full. To ensure that the resin runs freely, the collector should go home and drink a very hot cup of very thick corn *atole.*

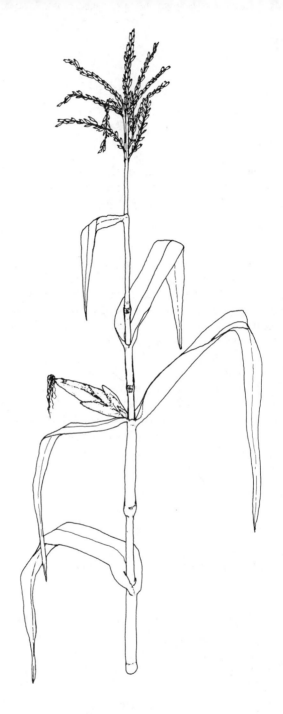

6 cm

Zea mays L.

CORN

Maize (E)
Maíz (S)
Ix-im (M)

Scientific Name: *Zea mays* L.

Plant Family: Poaceae

Description: An annual, cultivated plant growing to 2 m tall; leaves to 1 m long and drooping; flowers on terminal panicles, whitish; seeds formed in spikelets on a woody axis commonly known as "ears"; plant and spikelets extremely variable in size, habit, and color.

Habitat: A cultivated plant.

Traditional Uses: An excellent remedy for urinary conditions such as *retained urine, burning urine, kidney stones, bladder infections, gonorrhea,* and as a *lymphatic system cleanser* -- boil corn silk (the fine hairs) from 3 ears of corn in 3 cups water for 5 minutes and drink in sips all day long. Boil dry corn in water for 20 minutes and drink for treatment of *measles*.

Many indigenous people of Central America believe that maize is the "food of the Gods," given to humankind as a benediction. Another belief is that people were created from corn by the Gods.

Research Results: The silk is known to contain monoterpenes, a small amount of alkaloids, saponins, polyphenols, salicylic acid, tannins, allantoin, and salts of potassium (Hegnauer 1963; Flath et al. 1978; Paris & Moyse 1981; Ayensu 1982 -- cited in Robineau 1991).

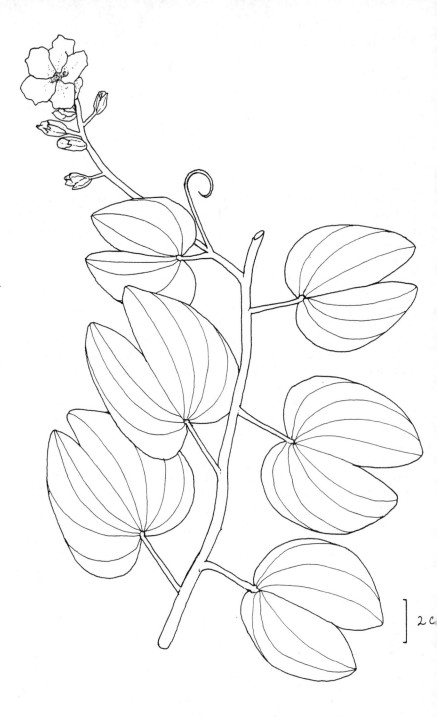

2 c

Bauhinia herrerae (Britt. & Rose) Standl. & Steyerm.

COWFOOT VINE

Pata de Vaca (S)
Ki-bix (M)

Scientific Name: *Bauhinia herrerae* (Britt. & Rose) Standl. & Steyerm.

Plant Family: Caesalpiniaceae

Description: Woody vine to 50 m long, growing into the canopy; leaves green, in the shape of a cow's hoof (giving rise to the common name); flowers with orange-yellow petals, numerous and showy on the vine.

Habitat: Forests (especially in gaps and in disturbed areas) and roadsides.

Traditional Uses: The stem is used as an astringent to staunch *diarrhea* and *bleeding*, to reduce *hemorrhage*, and to wash *wounds*. Boil a handful of chopped vine in 3 cups of water for 10 minutes; allow to cool and drink 1/2 cup 6 times daily for *headaches*, *internal wounds*, and *bleeding*, or 2 cups in 1/2 hour for *hemorrhage*. Use this same decoction to wash bleeding or infected *wounds*. For *headaches*, mash a handful of leaves in 1 quart of water; place in sun for 1 hour and wash head with this water. The leaves are a component of some of the traditional bath mixtures used to treat many ailments.

This is an old remedy for *birth control* among Maya women, now apparently mostly forgotten. Prepared from a handful of vine that has been boiled in 3 cups of water for 10 minutes, a cup is consumed before each meal all during the menstrual cycle. It is said that this dose is effective for up to 6 months. Drinking this decoction during 9 menstrual cycles is said to produce irreversible infertility in women.

According to Standley and Steyermark (1946), the Yucatec Maya have used the vine since ancient times for tying the crossbars and roof timbers of their houses. The bark is peeled from the stem, doubled over on its inner surface and stored in large rolls. For use, the rolls are wet and the bark becomes pliable enough to utilize for cordage.

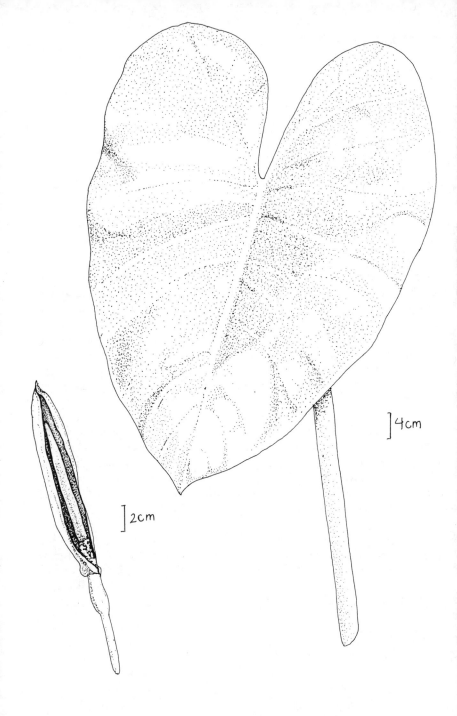

Alocasia macrorhiza (L.) G. Don.

CREOLE GAL

Carib Gal (E)
Wild Coco (E)

Scientific Name: *Alocasia macrorhiza* (L.) G. Don.

Plant Family: Araceae

Description: Herb to 1.5 m tall; leaves large, arrow-shaped, dark purple-green, growing from an underground bulb; flowers borne on spikes to 50 cm tall, with white bract enclosing creme-colored spadix.

Habitat: Clearings, yards, old fields; cultivated ornamental.

Traditional Uses: Boil 1 large leaf and stem in large pot of water for 10 minutes; use this as bath for *skin conditions* of all sorts (especially those that itch, or new burns). The fresh leaves can be made into a poultice and applied directly to *varicose veins* to improve circulation, prevent bursting, and reduce pain.

Hortus Third (Bailey and Bailey 1976) notes that the corms of this plant can be used for food (presumably only after proper preparation to eliminate the toxic compounds that may be contained in the plant). It is common in Belize to see this plant cultivated as an ornamental species around houses and in gardens. Due to the oxalates found in the fresh sap of this genus, caution is urged when using it on the skin or on mucous membranes.

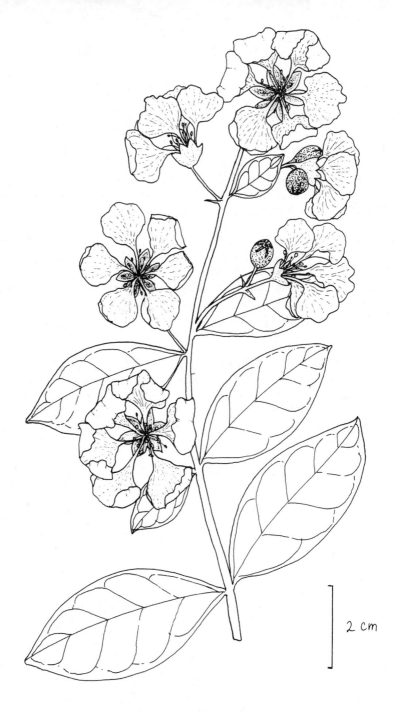

Lagerstroemia indica L.

CREPE MYRTLE

Scientific Name: *Lagerstroemia indica* L.

Plant Family: Lythraceae

Description: A shrub, sometimes a small tree, growing to 7 m tall; leaves oblong-elliptic to rounded, 2-7 cm long; inflorescences in panicles with white, yellow or purple flowers; fruit a capsule 9-13 mm long.

Habitat: Cultivated as an ornamental plant on farms and in public squares (plazas).

Traditional Uses: As a *diuretic*, boil 2 leaves in 3 cups water for 10 minutes and take in sips all day -- not to exceed 6 cups weekly. Boil a slice of bark 7.5 cm x 2.5 cm in 2 quarts of water for 10 minutes and use to bathe *wounds* and *infections*.

Research Results: An 80% ethanol extract of the freeze-dried, entire plant was tested and evaluated for antiviral activity against measles virus, adenovirus, Coxsackie B2 virus, herpes virus type 1, poliovirus 1, and Semlicki-Forest virus. All tests showed inactivity on the bark, with the exception of measles, the result of which was noted to be equivocal (Van Den Berghe et al. 1978). The leaf has been found to contain steroids (Goyal and Kumar 1987).

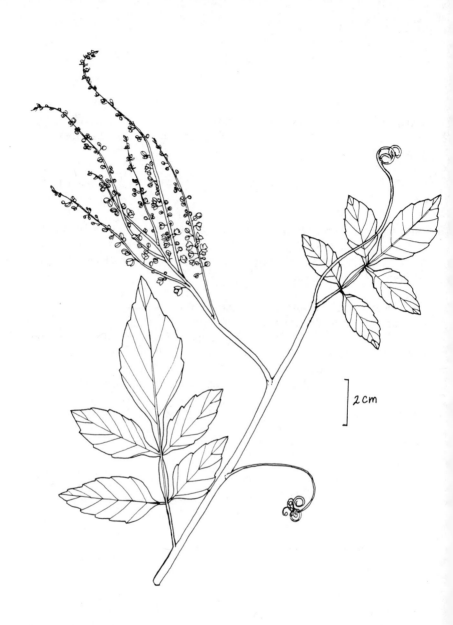

Paullinia tomentosa Jacq.

CROSS VINE

Skipping Rope Vine (E)
Cruxi (M)

Scientific Name: *Paullinia tomentosa* Jacq.

Plant Family: Sapindaceae

Description: Woody vine growing to 10 m tall; leaflets 10-20 cm long, serrate with small stipules; inflorescences developing from woody part of stem; flowers white, ca. 5 cm long; capsule ca. 2 cm long.

Habitat: Old fields, forests, trails.

Traditional Uses: These leaves are gathered alone or as part of an herbal formula containing 9 different medicinal leaves. Leaves are boiled to prepare bath for those suffering from a variety of complaints including *nervousness, sleeplessness, skin conditions, swellings, bruises,* and *burns.* Especially good to bathe babies who fall asleep on the cold cement floor and wake up with *aches* and *pains* -- mash leaves and stems in water, soak for 1 hour and heat.

Research Results: The plant is known to contain steroids and tannins (Domínguez S. and Alcorn 1985). A methanol extract of dried root was insecticidal against *Anostrepa ludens* at a concentration of 5 mg. Molluscicidal activity was shown from a methanol root extract in snails at a concentration of 50 PPM. Germination inhibition was shown in corn and beans from a 50 PPM extract of the root (ibid.).

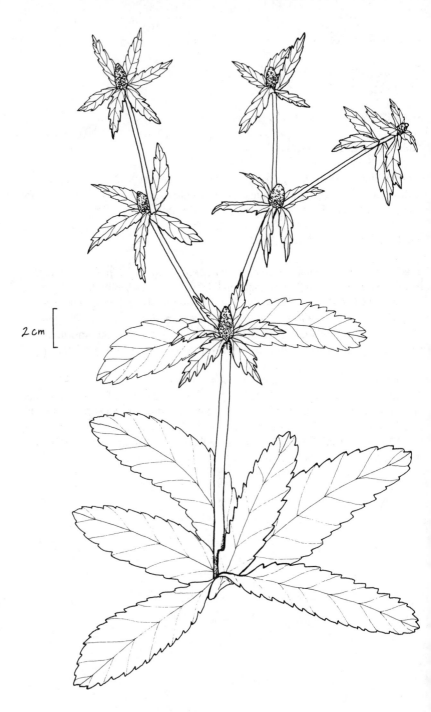

2 cm

Eryngium foetidum L.

CULANTRO (S)

Coriander (E)

Scientific Name: *Eryngium foetidum* L.

Plant Family: Apiaceae

Description: Perennial herb forming a low rosette of serrated leaves 8-20 cm long; leaves when crushed have a pleasant odor; flower stalk arising from center of rosette with several tight clusters of greenish white flowers surrounded by 5-6 bracts.

Habitat: Old fields, lawns, backyards, roadsides, sometimes cultivated.

Traditional Uses: Known as both food and medicine, the leaves are added to soups and stews giving a delightful taste to any dish, as well as to dispel *flatulence*. Drink as a tea to combat *stomach gas* or *indigestion*, and for *infantile vomiting* and *diarrhea*. To prepare tea, chop 6 leaves; pour boiling water over them and allow to steep for 15 minutes. Take in doses of 1/4 cup throughout the day.

As a condiment, add washed and chopped leaves to taste. Fresh, raw leaves may be added to salads.

Research Results: Anticonvulsant activity was demonstrated with a hot water extract of leaves and stems in mice at a dose of 3.0 ml (Simon and Singh 1986). A water extract of the entire plant, at a dose of 6.492 gm/kg, was shown to have antimalarial activity (*Plasmodium gallinaceum*) in chickens (Spencer et al. 1947).

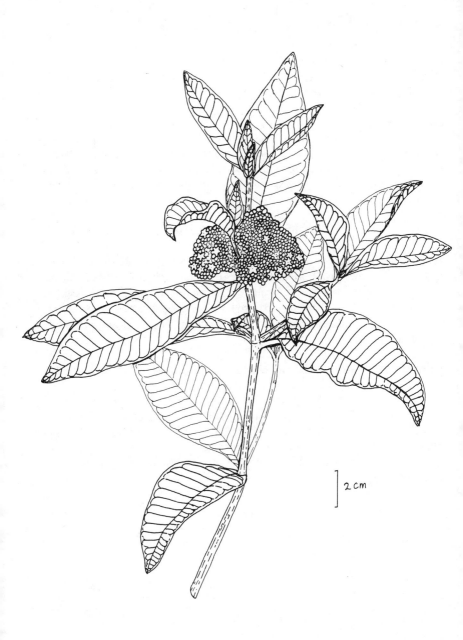

Psychotria tenuifolia Sw.

DOG'S TONGUE

Lengua de Perro (S)
X'Anal (M)

Scientific Name: *Psychotria tenuifolia* Sw.

Plant Family: Rubiaceae

Description: Shrub to 1 m tall; branches green and oblong-lanceolate; leaves 9-16 cm long and 1.5-5.5 cm wide; inflorescence a panicle, forming at the ends of the branches; flowers white, ca. 3 mm long; fruits bright red, globose, 4-5 mm in diameter.

Habitat: Forests.

Traditional Uses: Added to a mixture of medicinal leaves (usually 9) to make an herbal bath formula for bathing *wounds, rashes, swellings,* and for those who feel *nervous* and *sleepless.* Mash leaves and flowers to apply as poultice on *infected sores.*

This is the "male" Anal, the counterpart to the female Anal (*Psychotria acuminata*) discussed on page 11.

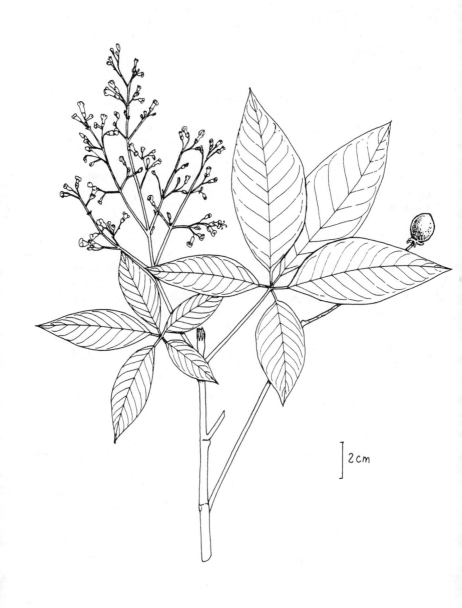

]2cm

Vitex gaumeri Greenm.

FIG TREE

Higuero (S)
Amate (M)

Scientific Name: *Ficus radula* Willd.

Plant Family: Moraceae

Description: Large tree up to 20 m, with a massive trunk that has a diameter up to 1 m; bark pale gray; roots vigorous, thick, visible on the trunk at ground level; leaves oval, pointed, dark green, shiny, 8-16 cm long; flowers whitish-pink; fruits pale green, containing pink flesh with many seeds.

Habitat: Riversides.

Traditional Uses: The white sap which oozes from stems and leaves of this tree is applied to *skin fungus, ringworm,* and *boils* 3 times daily. For *backache,* dampen a thin cotton cloth with latex of the fig tree and apply as poultice to painful area, placing a brown paper bag over cloth. Use bath of leaves to improve *circulation* in children and adults. To remove rotten, painful *teeth,* collect a small amount of white latex on a cotton ball and stuff inside tooth -- said to help remove tooth within the hour by breaking it into pieces and softening the flesh around the root.

The fruits, though dry and seedy, are edible.

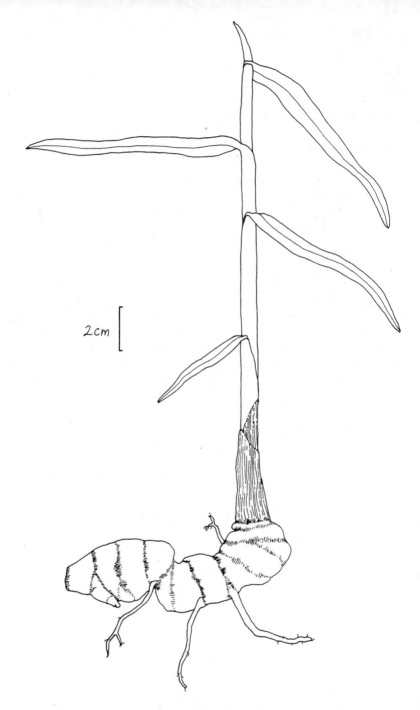

2cm

Zingiber officinale Roscoe

GINGER

Gengibre (S)

Scientific Name: *Zingiber officinale* Roscoe

Plant Family: Zingiberaceae

Description: Herbaceous plant to 1 m tall, growing from a fleshy, tuberous rhizome; leaves numerous, to 20 cm long by 2 cm wide; flowers pale green to greenish yellow, ca. 2 cm long, with purplish, yellow-dotted calyx lobe, on spikes ca. 5 cm long, rarely seen.

Habitat: Cultivated in gardens.

Traditional Uses: Grate 1 teaspoon of fresh ginger root in 1 cup of water; boil for 5 minutes and drink -- for *stomachache, gas pains, indigestion,* and *colds,* this household remedy offers great relief. For quick relief of *digestive upsets, nausea,* and *vomiting,* including car or air sickness, simply chew on a slice of fresh ginger. For *chest colds,* and *muscle aches and pains,* soak a cotton or flannel cloth in hot ginger tea made from chopped, boiled root and apply hot over area; cover with towels and repeat 6 times. For *delayed labor,* sip hot ginger tea during delivery. For *menstrual pain,* apply grated ginger to warm towel and place over abdomen for 1 hour. For *bronchitis,* add honey to grated ginger and apply as poultice to the chest. Drink a tea of grated root as a *stimulant* beverage in place of coffee or tea.

Research Results: Clinical studies have shown that capsules of ginger root can prevent motion sickness, as well as diarrhea and vomiting caused by gastrointestinal influenza (Mowrey and Clayson, 1982).

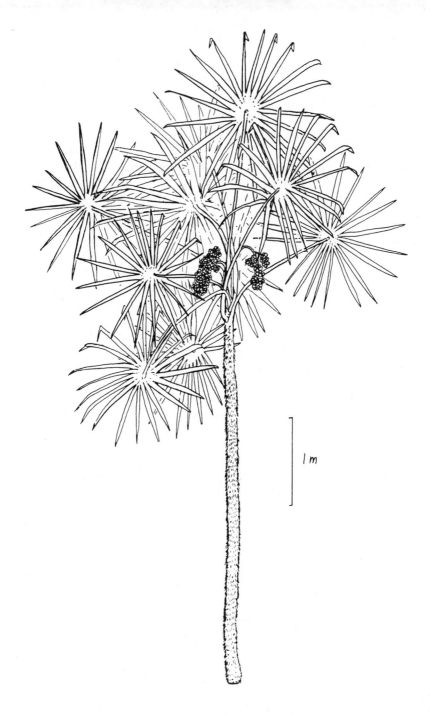

Crysophila argentea Bartlett

GIVE AND TAKE (C)

Escoba (S)

Scientific Name: *Crysophila argentea* Bartlett

Plant Family: Arecaceae

Description: Palm to 8 m tall; trunk to 10 cm in diameter, heavily spined; spines to 4 cm long; leaves numerous, palmate, glossy green above, silvery-white on underside; flowers creme-colored; fruits round, white, ca. 1.2 cm in diameter.

Habitat: Moist forests, both lowland and upland.

Traditional Uses: Its Creole name of "Give and Take" refers to the fact that this palm can give a very bad stinging cut from the thorns, but one can take a remedy for bleeding, infection, and pain from the inner portion of the leaf sheath and petiole. The inside part of the sheath and petiole is pink, cotton-like and sticky. It is applied to fresh wounds to *staunch bleeding, prevent infection*, and *alleviate pain*.

Brooms are made from young, dried leaves tied together on a slender stick.

Research Results: Alkaloids were found to be present in the leaf (Domínguez S. et al. 1962).

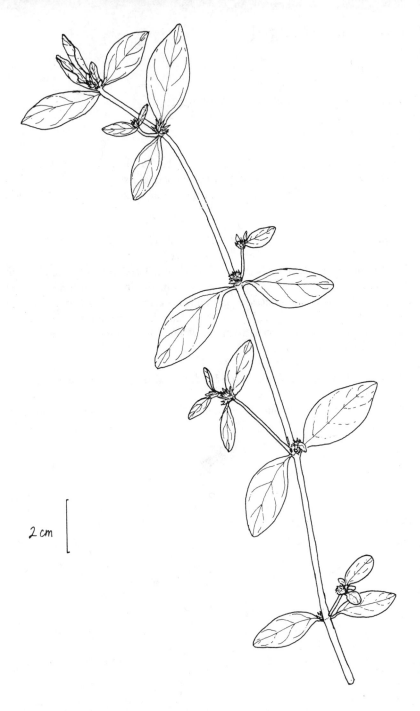

2 cm

Alternanthera flavogrisea Urb.

GOLONDRINA (S)

Xix-can-lol (M)

Scientific Name: *Alternanthera flavogrisea* Urb.

Plant Family: Amaranthaceae

Description: Low growing plant to 40 cm tall, running along ground; stems woody; leaves lanceolate, to 5 cm long x 1.5 cm wide; flowers green-white.

Habitat: Clearings, yards, roadsides.

Traditional Use: This common weed has long served as a household remedy for *flu, colds, urinary conditions, tiredness, postpartum tonics, granulated eyes, headaches, diabetes, fevers, internal infections* (especially of reproductive organs; for example, *inflammation of the ovaries*), and for those "who eat too much salt." Boil a handful -- about 1 entire fresh plant -- in 3 cups water for 2 minutes; drink 1 cup before meals 3 times daily.

Juice of fresh, mashed leaves is a good poultice to *staunch bleeding* or use as mouthwash to treat *mouth sores* and *thrush*.

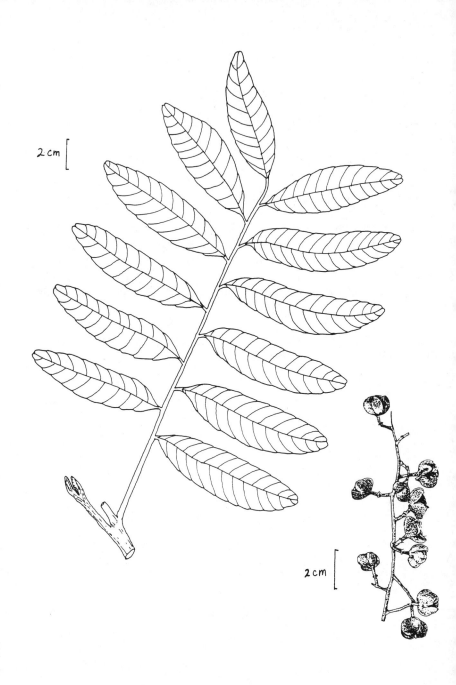

2 cm

2 cm

Cupania belizensis Standl.

GRANDE BETTY

Palo Carbón (S)
Chac-pom (M)

Scientific Name: *Cupania belizensis* Standl.

Plant Family: Sapindaceae

Description: Tree to 12 m or more, with trunk to 30 cm in diameter; leaflets shiny green above, with small hairs on undersides; inflorescences much branched; capsules 3-lobed; seeds shiny black and yellow.

Habitat: Moist primary and secondary forests, and in clearings.

Traditional Uses: The trunk is used to make charcoal, hence the Spanish name "palo carbon." The leaves are used as an herbal bath for *sprains, bruises*, and *swellings* -- wash the affected part with a cooled decoction of leaves 3 times daily until it gets better. For "*bad belly*" or *diarrhea*, boil a piece of bark 2.5 x 8 cm in 3 cups water for 10 minutes and take in sips all day, avoiding cold foods or drinks.

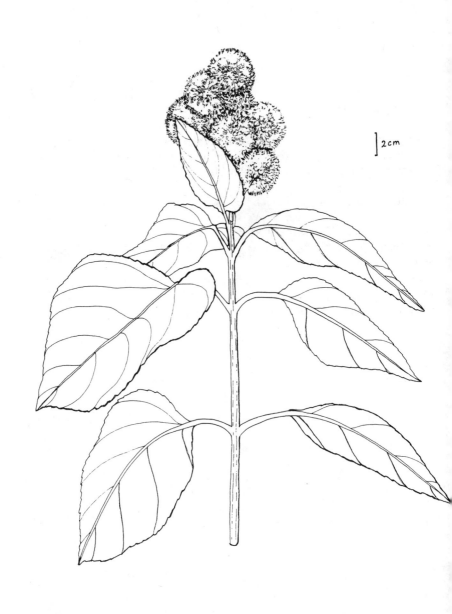

]2cm

Eupatorium (Critonia) morifolium Mill.

GREEN STICK

Palo Verde (S)
Xa-ax-como-che (M)

Scientific Name: *Eupatorium (Critonia) morifolium* Mill.

Plant Family: Asteraceae

Description: Herbaceous shrub, growing to 4 m tall; stems thick, green, hollow, often woody; leaves opposite with toothed margins, 10-40 cm in length; flowers greenish-yellow, turning straw-brown when dry.

Habitat: Forest, edge of forests, riversides, roadsides.

Traditional Uses: Of the medicinal leaves found in the forest, this is one of the most important and useful to add to herbal bath formulas. Steam baths ("bajos") are given in cases of *swelling, retention of fluids, rheumatism, arthritis, paralysis*, and *muscle spasms*. The leaf is heated in oil and applied to *boils, tumors, cysts*, and *pus-filled sores*. Boil leaf alone or in combination with other bathing leaves for any *skin condition, exhaustion, wounds, feverish babies, insomnia, flu, aches, pains*, and *general malaise*.

Research Results: There is little chemical or pharmacological information about this plant. Martinez (1984) noted that a decoction of the dried leaf, root, and twig was used to treat wounds and bruises in Puebla, Mexico.

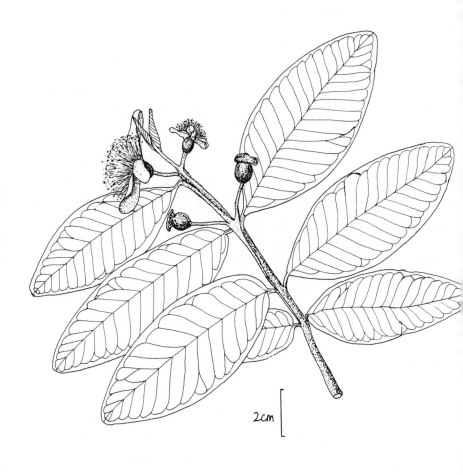

2cm

Psidium guajava L.

GUAVA

Guayaba (S)
Pici (M)

Scientific Name: *Psidium guajava* L.

Plant Family: Myrtaceae

Description: Tree growing to 10 m tall; stem slender, smooth with variously colored light and dark brown bark; leaves 8-14 cm long x 3-6 cm wide, somewhat leathery; flowers at ends of branches, with white petals, ca. 1-1.5 cm long; stamens numerous (to 275), white; fruit rounded, 2-6 cm long, yellow or pink when ripe.

Habitat: Edge of forests, old fields, roadsides.

Traditional Uses: Infuse 1 cup of green leaves in 3 cups boiling water for 20 minutes and gargle 2 times daily for *mouth sores, bleeding* from the *gums*, or as a *douche* for *leukorrhea* and relaxed walls of the vagina *after childbirth*. Chewing on tender leaves is an old remedy for *bleeding gums* and *bad breath*, and is said to allay *hangovers* if chewed before drinking.

Boil 9 leaves and 9 young fruits in 3 cups water for 10 minutes; drink 1 cup warm before meals 3 times daily for *diarrhea, dysentery, upset stomach*, and *colds*. Mashed or pounded (macerated) flowers are applied as a poultice to painful conditions of the eye due to *sun strain, conjunctivitis*, or *accident*. A tea made from the bark, which is rich in astringent tannins, is an excellent remedy for *diarrhea, vomiting, upset stomach, dysentery, sore throat*, and as a wash for *wounds* and *ulcers* of the skin -- boil a strip of bark 2.5 cm wide x 5 cm long in 3 cups of water for 10 minutes; drink 1 cup before meals. To bathe *sores* on skin, boil young leaves and flowers; toast leaves and flowers to a powder and sprinkle on sores after bath.

Research Results: A hot water extract of dried leaf was shown to have *in vitro* activity against *Sarcina lutea, Staphylococcus aureus*, and *Mycobacterium phlei* (Malcom and Sofowora 1969). A hot water extract of dried leaf showed hyperglycemic activity in mice at a dose of 5 gm/kg, with a 16% rise in blood sugar (Mueller-Oerlinghausen et al. 1971). Antifungal activity was demonstrated using a fresh leaf water extract at an unspecified concentration against *Ustilago maydis* amd *Ustilago nuda* (Singh and Pathak 1984). One guava has 2-5 times more Vitamin C than does an orange (Purseglove 1974).

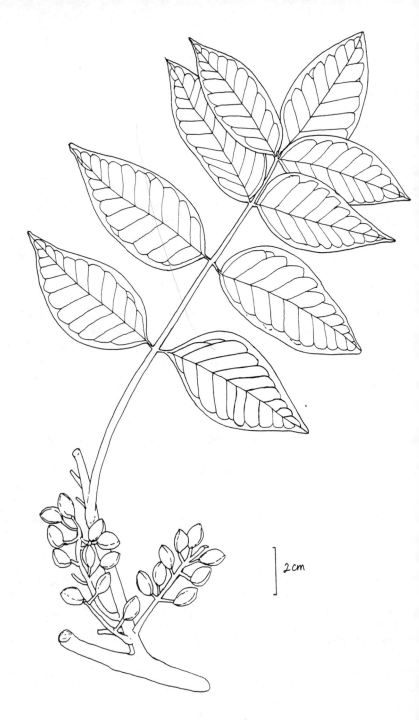

2 cm

Bursera simaruba (L.) Sarg.

GUMBOLIMBO

Indio Desnudo (S)
Cha-cah (M)

Scientific Name: *Bursera simaruba* (L.) Sarg.

Plant Family: Burseraceae

Description: Tree to 25 m tall with characteristic red, shaggy bark which peels off in paper thin strips; branchlets shiny; leaves deciduous with 5-7 leaflets, each 5-12 cm long; flowers greenish or yellowish, fragrant; fruit round, 6-10 mm long, tinged with red.

Habitat: Common in primary and disturbed forests; also used as living fence posts.

Traditional Uses: *Antidote* to poisonwood sap which causes blistering, swelling, itching, and severe discomfort -- peel bark from tree and boil a strip 2.5-5 cm x 30 cm in 1 gallon of water for 10 minutes; cool and use to bathe affected area 3 times daily. This bark bath will also alleviate the discomfort of *insect bites, sunburn, rashes, skin sores*, and *measles*. Drink same bath preparation as tea for *internal infections,* to *purify blood*, for *urinary tract conditions, fevers, sun stroke, colds, flu*; wrap forehead with leaves to reduce *headaches*. A steam bath of the leaves is said to be useful against *typhoid*; the patient should also lie on a bed of leaves. For *kidney ailments* or *pain*, boil a piece of bark 15 cm x 30 cm in 3 quarts of water for 10 minutes and drink all day in place of water -- this treatment is said to cleanse kidneys and remove any infection that may be present.

Research Results: A methanol extract of the dried bark of gumbolimbo was found to have molluscicidal activity against snails and inhibited germination in beans (Domínguez S. and Alcorn 1985).

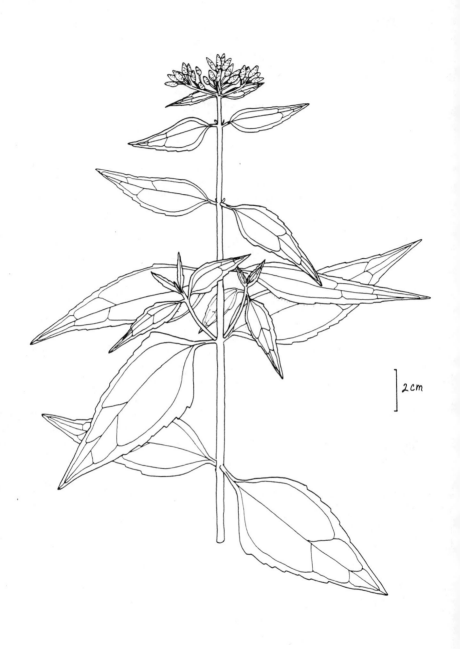

Chromolaena odorata (L.) K. & R.

HATZ (M)

Jack-in-Bush (C)

Scientific Name: *Chromolaena odorata* (L.) K. & R.

Plant Family: Asteraceae

Description: Shrub to 1-2 m tall or more, with many branches; leaves strongly aromatic; flowers in clusters of 20-35, flat-topped, lavender or white; seeds black.

Habitat: Fields, pastures, forest margins, disturbed sites.

Traditional Uses: Boil leaves to use as herbal bath for many ailments, but especially as analgesic for *headaches* and *pain*; also for *nervousness* and *insomnia*. For baths, boil double handful of leaves in 1 gallon water. Bathe head with cooled decoction if headaches occur during daylight hours or with hot decoction if headaches occur after nightfall.

Boil 9 branchlets with leaves in 3 cups of water for 5 minutes. Drink as a tea to *calm nerves* (sip hot throughout day), for *insomnia* (take one hot cup of tea 1 hour before bedtime), for *depression*, and for *coughs* and *colds*.

Research Results: *In vitro* studies have shown antibacterial activity of dried leaves and stem against *Bacillus subtilis* (Avirutnant and Pongpan 1983); dried leaves showed coagulant activity in rats and a decrease in prothrombin time (Jiravanit et al. 1985); fresh leaf extract has shown *in vitro* antifungal activity against *Rhizopus* sp. and *Ustilago maydis* (Awuah 1989); and leaf essential oil has shown *in vitro* antibacterial activity against *Bacillus subtilis, Escherichia coli, Klebsiella aerogenes*, and *Staphylococcus aureus* (Inya-agha et al. 1987). Chemical evaluation of the plant has shown it to contain monoterpenes and sesquiterpenes (ibid.) and flavonoids (Barua et al. 1978).

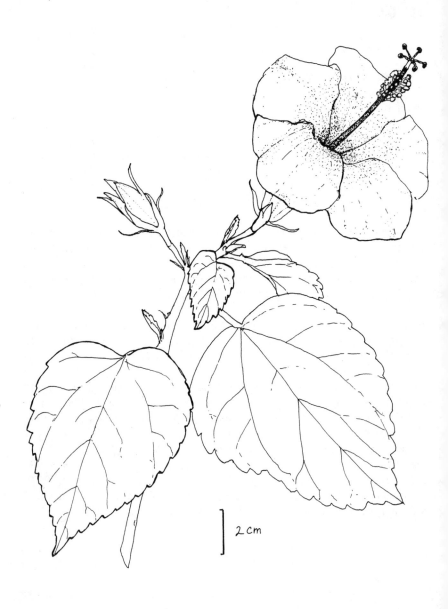

] 2 cm

Hibiscus rosa-sinensis L.

HIBISCUS

Tulipán (S)

Scientific Name: *Hibiscus rosa-sinensis* L.

Plant Family: Malvaceae

Description: A woody shrub growing to 8 m tall, with slender stems and many branches; flowers bright red with yellow stamen tubes.

Habitat: Cultivated in yards and naturalized along roadsides and old fields.

Traditional Uses: Only the red-flowered hibiscus is considered of medicinal value. For *post partum hemorrhages*, the *staunching of excessive menstrual flow*, and to *prevent miscarriage*, boil 9 leaves with 1 open and 1 closed flower in 3 cups of water for 10 minutes; drink warm. A cool bath of leaves and flowers is useful to treat various *skin conditions*. For *headaches* and *fevers*, mash leaves and apply to the head. The flowers are edible and rich in iron. They can be eaten to treat *painful menstruation*.

Research Results: An ethanol-water (1:1) extract of the aerial parts of this species showed central nervous system depressant activity in mice at a dose of 500 mg/kg (Bhakuni et al. 1969). Hypotensive activity in a dog was obtained using an ethanol-water (1:1) extract of the aerial parts at a dose of 50 mg/kg (ibid.). Numerous studies in the area of reproduction have been carried out with this plant. An embryotoxic effect was obtained from a water extract administered to female rats at an unspecified dose (Kholkute et al. 1976). Antiestrogenic effects in female rats obtained using various extracts at various dose levels are reported in Kholkute and Udupa (1976).

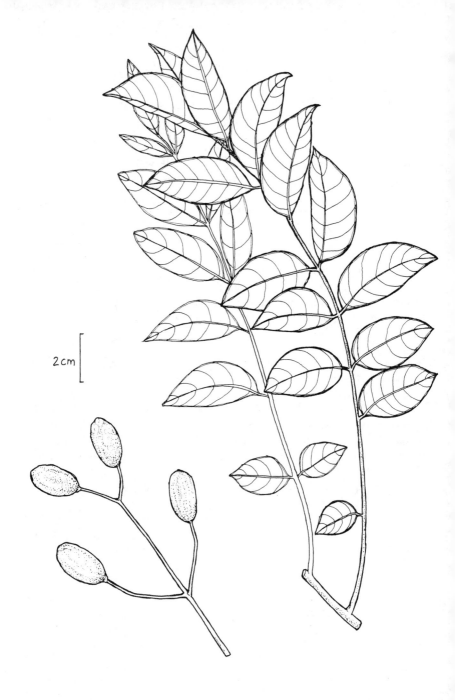

Spondias radlkoferi Donn. Sm.

HOG PLUM

Jobo (S)
Puk (M)

Scientific Name: *Spondias radlkoferi* Donn. Sm.

Plant Family: Anacardiaceae

Description: Tree growing to 10 m with a stem diameter of 25 cm; leaves with 5-9 pairs of leaflets; flowers white, forming in large panicles, each flower to 3 mm long; fruits yellow, ovoid, ca. 3-4 cm long.

Habitat: Forests, roadsides, pastures.

Traditional Uses: Drink as an astringent tea for *diarrhea, gonorrhea,* or *sore throat* -- boil a handful of flower buds and bark together in 3 cups water for 10 minutes; drink 1 cup before each meal. For *gonorrhea,* take in this way for 10 days and re-test. Use as a bath for stubborn *sores, rashes,* painful *insect stings,* and to bathe *pregnant women* who feel *weak* and *tired* beyond first trimester -- boil a large double handful of leaves and a strip of bark 3 cm x 15 cm in 2 gallons of water for 10 minutes.

Research Results: A closely related species (*Spondias mombin*) has shown *in vitro* antibacterial activity using a 95% ethanol extract at concentrations of 10% (*Escherichia coli, Micrococcus luteus, Pseudomonas aeruginosa,* and *Shigella dysenteriae*) and 5% (*Salmonella typhosa, Shigella dysenteriae,* and *Staphylococcus aureus*); using water extracts at a concentration of 20%, activity was shown against *Escherichia coli, Micrococcus luteus, Pseudomonas aeruginosa, Salmonella typhosa,* and *Staphylococcus aureus* (Ajao et al. 1985). Antiviral activity from ethanol (100%) extracts of leaf and stem was shown against Coxsackie B4 virus, *Herpes simplex,* and *poliovirus* (unspecified) (Corthout et al. 1985). Uterine stimulant effect was obtained in rats using a water extract (Barros et al. 1970).

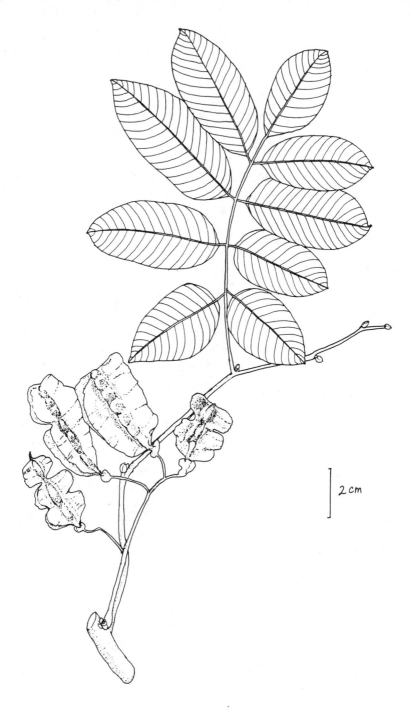

2 cm

Piscidia piscipula (L.) Sarg.

JABIN (S)

Palo de Gusano (S)
Dogwood, May Bush (E)

Scientific Name: *Piscidia piscipula* (L.) Sarg.

Plant Family: Fabaceae

Description: Large shrub or tree to 15 m tall; stem to 30 cm, grayish, with rough bark; leaflets 9-13, each 4-8 cm long; flowers pink or white and red, in panicles 8-20 cm long; fruits green, 2-7.5 cm long x 2-4 cm wide, each containing 1-6 seeds.

Habitats: Forests.

Traditional Uses: Boil a 5 x 5 cm square of bark in 3 cups of water for 10 minutes; drink for *diarrhea, dysentery, excessive menstruation*, and to *wash wounds, rashes*, and *skin conditions*. The same decoction is a good astringent and is used as a mouthwash for *bleeding gums*.

Research Results: A water extract of dried bark and root of this plant has shown antiviral activity in cell culture at a 10% concentration against poliovirus II, herpes virus type 2, influenza virus A2 [Manheim 57] and Vaccinia virus (May and Willuhn 1978). Antifungal activity in broth culture was shown using a hot water extract of dried leaves against *Epidermophyton floccosum, Microsporum canis, Microsporum gypseum, Trichophyton mentagrophytes*, and *Trichophyton rubrum* (Cáceres et al. 1991). Uterine relaxant effect in guinea pigs was shown using a 1-2 M concentration fluid extract of the plant and a hot water extract (Pilcher 1916). Root and bark extract with chloroform at a concentration of 1-99 M showed strong uterine relaxant effect in rats as did an ethanol extract (95%) (Butler and Mullen 1955). Molluscicidal activity using a methanol extract of dried wood (concentration of 50 PPM) was shown against snails (Domínguez S. and Alcorn 1985).

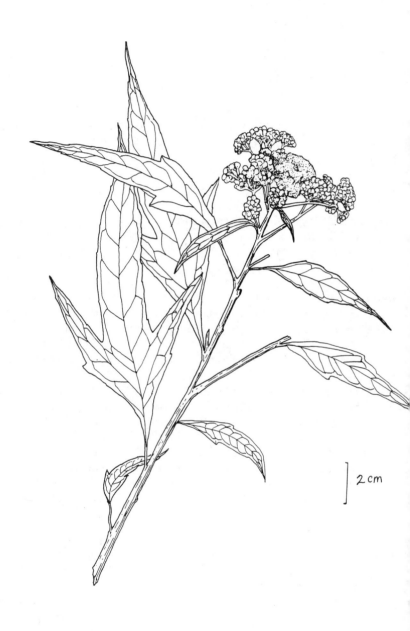

］ 2 cm

Neurolaena lobata (L.) R.Br.

JACKASS BITTERS

Tres Puntas, Mano de Lagarto (S)
Kayabim (M)

Scientific Name: *Neurolaena lobata* (L.) R.Br.

Plant Family: Asteraceae

Description: Herb growing to 1-4 m tall, with few main stems and numerous branches on each stem; leaves often with 3 distinctive points (hence the Spanish name), bitter tasting; flowers yellow.

Habitat: Clearings, roadsides, fields, pastures.

Traditional Uses: Entire plant is a highly respected medicinal used to treat and prevent a variety of parasitic ailments such as *malaria, fungus, ringworm, amoebas, intestinal parasites*, and boring organisms such as *beef worm* or *screwworm*. Tea is an excellent vaginal douche for *leukhorrea* and *itching*, and to bathe stubborn *wounds* or *infections*; it is also used to wash hair to kill *head lice*. Boiled, strained leaves can be used as *insecticide* or *fungicide* on diseased plants in house or garden. Leaves are toasted and powdered to use as wound powder applied directly to *sores, fungus*, and *infections*. Roots are boiled and drunk as *blood cleanser*. For teas, boil fresh leaf for each cup of water for 10 minutes; drink 1-3 cups daily for intestinal parasites. For baths, use one handful of leaves boiled to one gallon of water for 10 minutes; cool to warm and bathe area. Fresh juice from crushed leaves may be applied directly to *wounds, sores*, and *skin conditions* such as *fungus*.

Research Results: There is surprisingly little information about this plant in the pharmacological literature, relative to its importance in folk medicine. An ethanol extract (100%) demonstrated antihyperglycemic activity in mice at an oral dose of 250 mg/kg, and at a dose of 500 mg/kg demonstrated hypoglycemic activity in mice (Gupta et al. 1984). The leaves are known to contain sesquiterpenes (Manchand and Blount 1978) and flavonoids (Kerr et al. 1981).

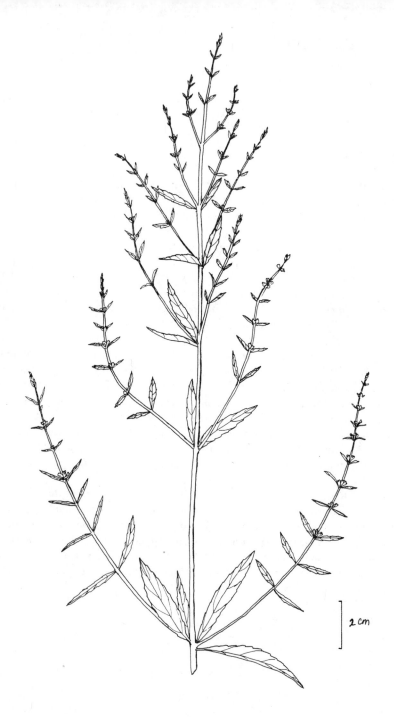

Hyptis verticillata Jacq.

JOHN CHARLES

Hierba Martín (S)

Scientific Name: *Hyptis verticillata* Jacq.

Plant Family: Lamiaceae

Description: Shrub with many branches, growing to 1-2 m tall; stems woody, usually square (especially when young); leaves dark green, small, pointed, aromatic; flowers small, greenish.

Habitat: Backyards, pastures, roadsides.

Traditional Uses: For *coughs, colds, mucus conditions, asthma onset, fever, tonsillitis, uterine fibroids,* and *bronchitis* -- steep small handful of leaves and branchlets in 3 cups water for 20 minutes; drink warm in 1/3 cup doses all day. Mix with lemon grass for high *fevers*. Boil entire plant to bathe children and infants with *malaise*. Add to gumbolimbo bark to bathe *contact dermatitis* of manchaneel tree. Boil and drink root for severe *gastric distress*. To relieve pain following *childbirth*, boil a small handful of plant material, either roots or leaves or both, in 3 cups of water for 10 minutes; drink 1 cup warm, 3 times daily before meals. Boil one entire plant in 1 gallon of water for 10 minutes to bath those with any sickness. In general, it is said that adding John Charles to any formula will give it added strength.

Research Results: An ethanol-water (1:1) extract of flower, leaves, and twigs exhibited *in vitro* cytotoxicity against 9KB cancer (National Cancer Institute 1976). A water extract of the plant exhibited *in vitro* cytotoxic activity against P-1534 leukemia (German 1971). Molluscicidal activity was obtained from a methanol extract at a concentration of 50 PPM in snails (Domínguez S. and Alcorn 1985). The leaf and stem of this plant contain the lignan podophyllotoxin (German 1971).

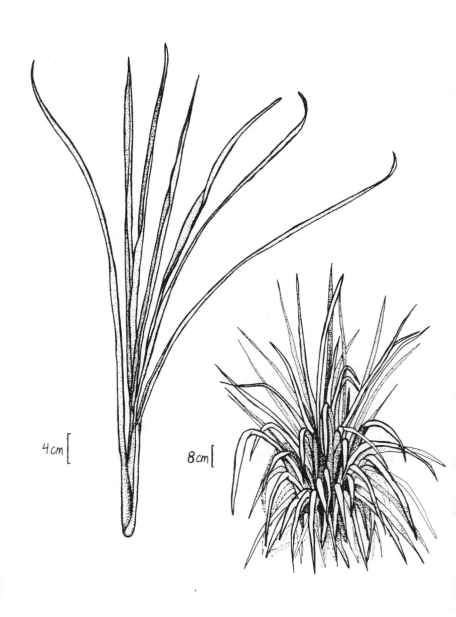

4cm [

8cm [

Cymbopogon citratus (DC.) Stapf

LEMON GRASS

Fever Grass (E)
Zacate Limón (S)

Scientific Name: *Cymbopogon citratus* (DC.) Stapf

Plant Family: Poaceae

Description: Perennial grass growing in dense tufts; leaves green, up to 2 m tall, producing a lemony aroma when crushed; rarely if ever producing flowers in cultivation.

Habitat: Cultivated in dooryard gardens.

Traditional Uses: Take as a tea for *fevers, coughs, colds*, and as a pleasant *tonic* or beverage. Promotes *perspiration* and *excretion of phlegm*, and eases *stomach cramps*. Especially useful for children and infants. For adult *fevers*, boil 1 mashed root and 10 leaves in 3 cups of water for 10 minutes; drink very hot; go to bed and wrap up warmly. For childhood *fevers*, boil 10 leaves in 3 cups of water for 10 minutes; give child 1/2 cup 6 times daily and keep child warm. Soak mashed root in oil and rub on *backache, muscle spasms*, and over forehead to relieve *headaches*.

Research Results: A great deal of research on bioactivity has been carried out on lemon grass. The essential oil extracted from fresh leaves and stems has shown *in vitro* antibacterial activity against *Staphylococcus aureus, Bacillus subtilis, Escherichia coli*, and *Pseudomonas aeruginosa* (Onawunmi and Ogunlana 1986). An extract of the dried entire plant showed *in vitro* antifungal activity against a variety of cultures (Soytong et al. 1985). The essential oil was shown to have *in vitro* activity against *Candida albicans, Candida pseudotropicalis*, and *Aspergillus fumigatus* (Onawunmi 1989). Hypothermic activity from a hot water extract of lemon grass was demonstrated in rats (Carlini et al. 1986), and the analgesic activity of the essential oil was demonstrated in mice and rats (Lorenzetti et al. 1991).

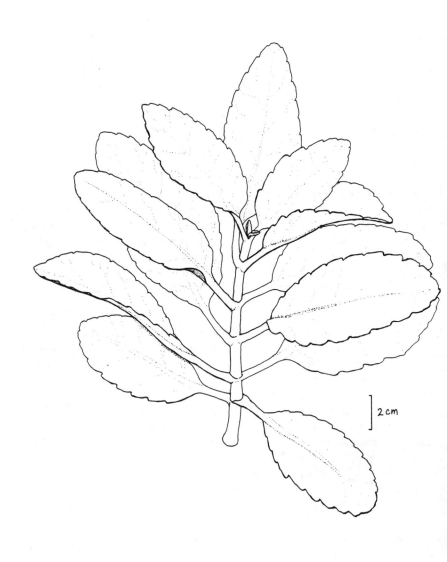

2 cm

Kalanchoe pinnata (Lam.) Pers.

LIFE EVERLASTING

Tree of Life (E)
Siempre Viva (S)

Scientific Name: *Kalanchoe pinnata* (Lam.) Pers.

Plant Family: Crassulaceae

Description: Fleshy herb to 1 m tall; leaves succulent, with scalloped edges; flowers showy, purplish-pink, trumpet-shaped, borne on tall panicles.

Habitat: Yards, home gardens, old fields.

Traditional Uses: Mash leaf and apply to forehead to relieve *headaches*; apply fresh to *bruises, swellings*, and *cuts*. Make decoction of leaves for *coughs, colds, sore throat, flu, weakness*, and to bathe *swellings, sprains*, and *bruises*. Mash leaves with castor oil and apply to breasts for *mastitis*. Leaf is eaten with salt for a variety of ailments. Said to be a panacea.

Called "Life Everlasting" because when leaves fall to ground new plants sprout from scalloped edges and take root.

Research Results: There have been a number of pharmacological studies carried out with this plant. A water extract of the fresh plant was shown to be cytotoxic against 9KB cancer in cell culture (Yamagishi et al. 1989). A hot water extract of dried leaf was shown to exhibit antifungal activity against *Trichophyton mentagrophytes*, a causal agent of athlete's foot (*Tinea pedis*) (Rai and Upadhyay 1988). Other antifungal activity was shown against *Ustilago maydis* and *U. nuda* (Singh and Pathak 1984). Anti-inflammatory activity was observed after a methanol extract in a dose of 300 mg/kg was administered to rats (Siddhartha and Chaudhuri 1990). Finally, a cautionary note is advised, based on the death of 2 calves fed fresh flowers at a rate of 20 gm/kg. The first died 9 hours after dosing, collapsing with dyspnea, tachycardia, and irregular heart rate. The second had diarrhea and tachycardia and died 15 hours after dosing. Emphysema was noted in one animal and both had focal myocardial degeneration (McKenzie et al. 1987). This species is rich in chemical compounds, with over two dozen identified.

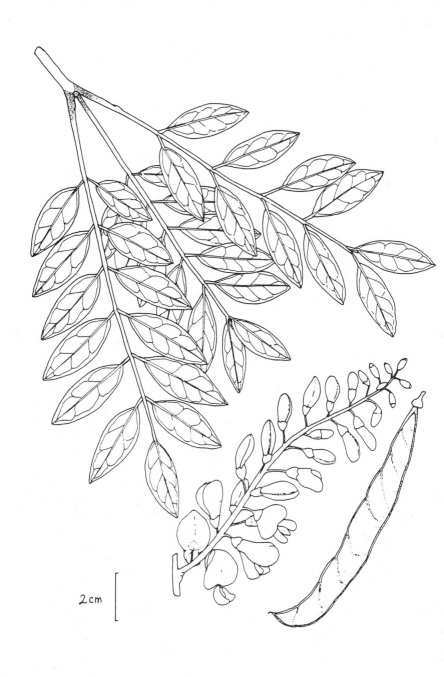

2cm

Gliricidia sepium (Jacq.) Steud.

106

MADRE DE CACAO (S)

Sayab (M)

Scientific Name: *Gliricidia sepium* (Jacq.) Steud.

Plant Family: Fabaceae

Description: A tree growing to 10 m high; trunk thin, to 30 cm in diameter; bark brown, somewhat rough; leaves deciduous, divided into 7-17 leaflets each 3-7 cm long; flowers bright pink to white, in dense, multiflowered racemes 5-10 cm long; pods dark brown, 10-15 cm long by 1-1.5 cm wide.

Habitat: Forests, fields, roadsides, planted as living fence posts.

Traditional Uses: Boiled, cooled bark water is useful for washing *tired, burning,* or *irritated eyes* -- slice a piece of bark 8 cm x 2.5 cm and boil in 1 cup of water for 10 minutes; strain through a cloth twice and use to wash eyes. Seeds and bark are pulverized and mixed with ground corn to kill rats. Mash fresh leaves and apply as poultice for *wounds, ulcers, boils,* and *diaper rash.*

In Mexico, an excellent brown soap known as Cacahuananche is made from the bark. It is suitable for washing hair, skin, and laundry. The fresh flowers are eaten as a vegetable, primarily when cooked with eggs. According to Standley and Steyermark (1946), cattle feed on the leaves, which are toxic to rodents and dogs.

Research Results: Aerial parts of Madre de Cacao in a 1:1 ethanol-water extract were shown to have anti-inflammatory activity in rats at a dose of 0.375 mg/kg (Dhawan et al. 1977). Insecticidal activity of petroleum ether extracts of leaf, flowers, fruit, and root was observed against *Aedes aegypti* (yellow fever mosquito) (Sievers et al. 1949). Chemical analysis of the plant yielded flavonoids and carbohydrates (Dayal 1985) and proteids (Lavin 1986).

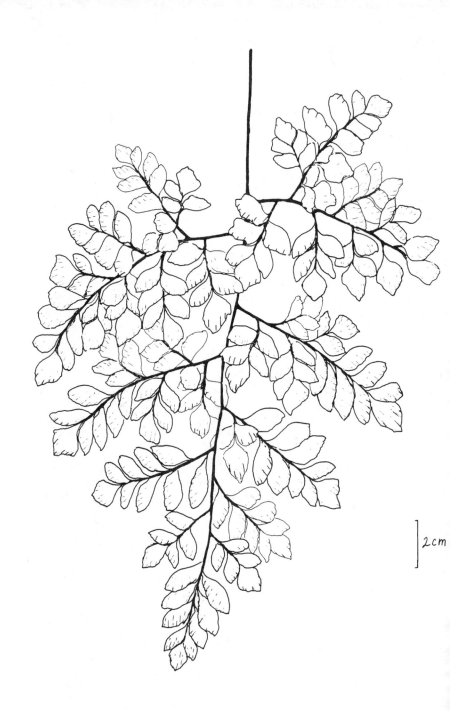

Adiantum tenerum Sw.

MAIDEN HAIR FERN

Black Stick (E)
Helecho, Palo Negro (S)
Ok-pich, Ek-chi-chan (M)

Scientific Name: *Adiantum tenerum* Sw.

Plant Family: Polypodiaceae

Description: A delicate fern to 30-50 cm tall; leaves with small, fan-shaped pinnae and black, brittle stems; sori brown, squarish or oblong, placed along edges of pinnae.

Habitat: Riversides, wet places, forests, rocky outcroppings.

Traditional Uses: For *coughs*, as an *expectorant*, and as an aid to *detoxification* of alcoholics -- steep 3 stems with leaves in 3 cups boiling water for 20 minutes and drink in sips all day. This tea will also increase production of *mother's milk*, aid *kidney function*, and has *antiparasitic* activity. Apply macerated leaves to scalp to get rid of *dandruff*. In Cuba and Argentina, a tea from the leaf is used to promote *menstrual discharge* (Martinez-Crovetto 1981; Roig y Mesa 1945).

This plant is said to have been used by the ancient Maya to decorate ceremonial altars.

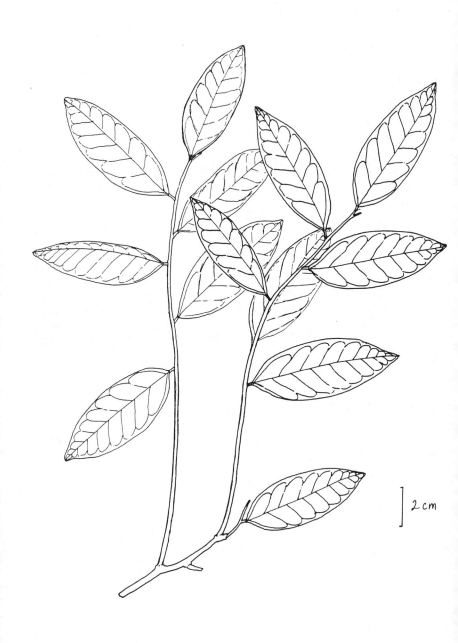

]2 cm

Agonandra sp.

110

MAN VINE

Bejuco de Hombre, Bejuco Verde (S)
Ya-ax-ak (M)

Scientific Name: *Agonandra* sp.

Plant Family: Olacaceae

Description: Vine growing to 15 m high and 10 cm in diameter; leaves small, opposite, oval-shaped; inner vine is ringed with whorls much like a tree; flower unknown.

Habitat: Forests (only on hillsides).

Traditional Uses: Chop woody part of vine; boil a small handful in 3 cups of water for 10 minutes and drink 1 cup before each meal for *constipation, intestinal gas, indigestion, mucus in stool, inability to eat* even a small portion of food, *gastritis*, and any ailment to do with the *digestive* or *alimentary tract*. This same tea also acts as an excellent mild *sedative*, and can be drunk for *backaches, neckache, headaches, muscle spasms*, and for males who pass *mucus in the urine*. The root is a superior remedy for male *impotency* -- chop root and boil 1 small handful in 3 cups of water for 10 minutes; drink 1 cup before each meal. Note that while drinking man vine tea, one must abstain from all acid foods, cold drinks, and beef.

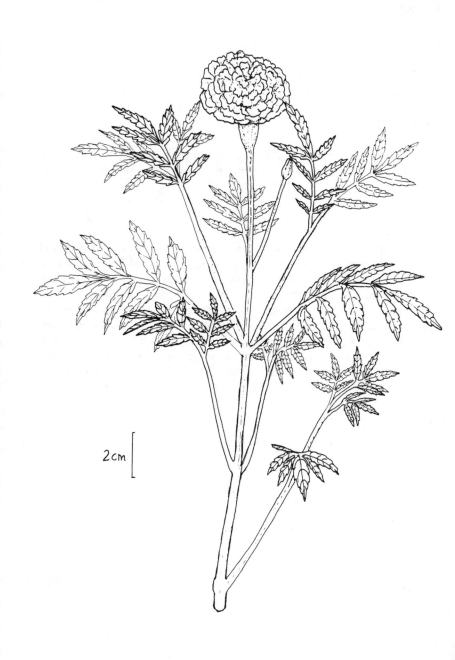

Tagetes erecta L.

MARIGOLD

Flor de Muerto (S)
Ix-ti-pu (M)

Scientific Name: *Tagetes erecta* L.

Plant Family: Asteraceae

Description: Erect annual herb to 1 m tall; leaves pinnate, aromatic; flowers in solitary heads, to 5 cm across, yellow to gold, aromatic.

Habitat: Pastures, old fields, yards, patios.

Traditional Uses: This plant is a *stimulant* and *perspiration producer.* Steep 3 flowers in 1 cup of hot boiled water for 10 minutes and drink to relieve *fever, infant colic, gastric pains, flatulence,* and *headaches.* A branch of the leaves is used to hold over pulse of infants while saying healing *prayers* ("ensalmos"). Boil entire plant in 2 gallons water for 10 minutes and bathe infants and young children suffering from *malaise, colic, diarrhea, fever, colds,* and *flu.* Use same decoction to bathe *sores, abscesses, cuts, wounds,* etc. Bunches of the flowers are hung in houses to keep out bats.

Garinagu people make a mixture of orange peel and marigold flowers to get rid of evil spirits. Funeral attendants wash hands in water in which the flowers have been soaked.

During Maya ceremonies, the priest washes his hands and face with a decoction of leaves and flowers to be better able to call the spirits.

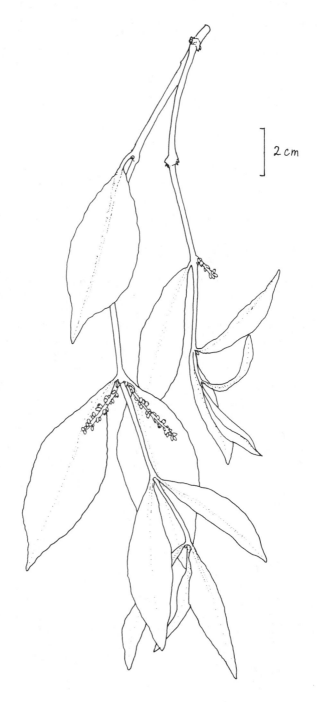

Phoradendron piperoides (HBK.) Trel.

MATAPALO (S)

Scorn the Earth, God Almighty Bush (E)

Scientific Name: *Phoradendron piperoides* (HBK.) Trel.

Plant Family: Loranthaceae

Description: Small parasitic shrub, erect or hanging, forming dense masses on host plants; leaves 5-12 cm long x 1.5-7 cm wide; flowers in spikes 2.5-6 cm long, yellow-green; fruit yellow-orange or brown, 5 mm long.

Habitat: Found growing as a parasite on trees, particularly on citrus, mango, and avocado.

Traditional Uses: Boil entire plant in water for 10 minutes and use warm as a wash for *skin conditions, infections, swellings*, and *bruises*. Mash with garlic and apply as a poultice to treat *dog bites*.

Research Results: Very little work has been carried out on this species. It was shown to have a contracting effect (non-specific) in guinea pigs using a hot water extract at a concentration of 0.5 mg/ml (Queiroz Neto and Melito 1990). A toxic effect was obtained in mice using a 2% acetic acid extract at an unspecified dose; the toxic effect was later shown to be due to protein (Samuelsson et al. 1981). Two related species, *Phoradendron flavescens* (Pursh) Nutt. and *P. villosum* Nutt., are known as mistletoe in North America. The berries and leaves are considered toxic if ingested (Kingsbury, 1964).

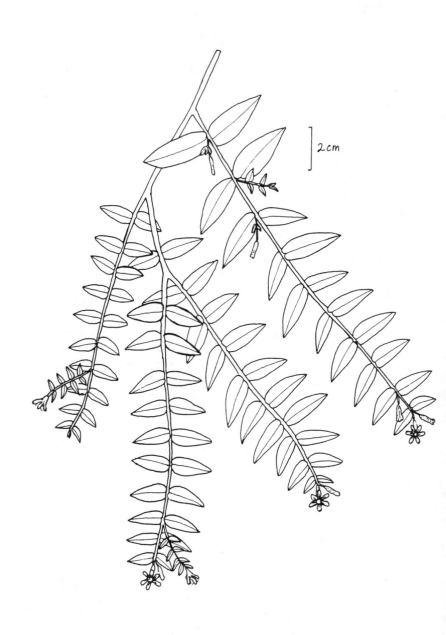

Cuphea calophylla Cham. & Schlecht.

MEXICAN HEATHER

Corriente, Corrimiento, Mañanita (S)
Schma-mo-cal (M)

Scientific Name: *Cuphea calophylla* Cham. & Schlecht.

Plant Family: Lythraceae

Description: Prostrate herb growing to 50 cm tall; leaves small; flowers tiny, mauve, borne on the ends of the branches.

Habitat: Old fields, edge of forests, trails, roadsides.

Traditional Uses: Boil entire plant to bathe those who feel *exhausted* or *chronically tired* and give 1 cup to drink with bath at bedtime. For *dysentery*, drink a decoction of entire plant until cured.

Research Results: Very little research has been carried out on this plant. An ethanol-water (50%) extract at a dose of 40 ml/kg showed diuretic activity in rats (Ribeiro et al. 1988). An ethanol-water (1:1) extract showed hypotensive activity in rats at a dose of 40 ml/kg (Ribeiro et al. 1986).

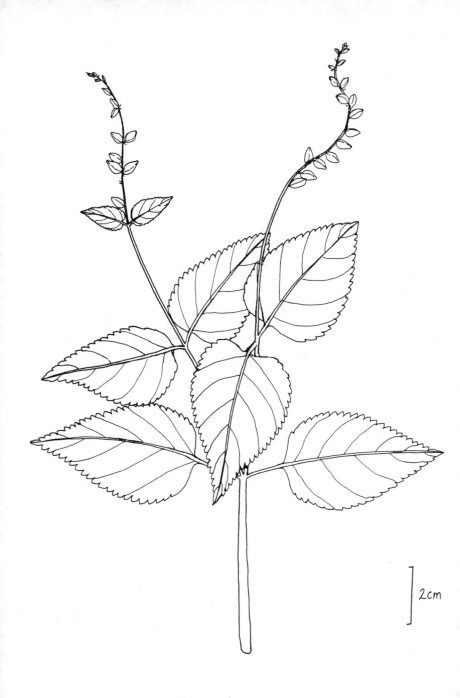

Priva lappulacea (L.) Pers.

118

MOSOTE (S)

Pega Ropa (S)

Scientific Name: *Priva lappulacea* (L.) Pers.

Plant Family: Verbenaceae

Description: Annual herb to 75 cm tall; leaves hairy, 2-10 cm long; flowers light purple, in racemes 5-20 cm long; fruits green, turning brown when mature.

Habitat: Yards, fields, doorsteps.

Traditional Uses: For *internal parasites*, boil a handful of leaves in 3 cups of water for 10 minutes; drink 3 cups of tea daily for 3 days, followed by a purge. Leaves parched over a flame are powdered and applied to *sores, infections, wounds*, and *fungal conditions*. Mash leaves into a poultice and rub juice on *itching skin condition* or *rashes*.

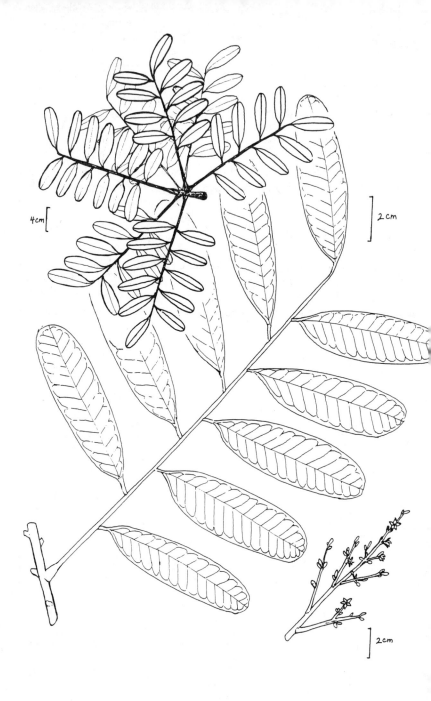

Simarouba glauca DC.

NEGRITO (S)

Dysentery Bark (E)
Pa-sak (M)

Scientific Name: *Simarouba glauca* DC.

Plant Family: Simaroubaceae

Description: Tree growing to 20 m tall; branches many, long, crooked, with stem diameter up to 30 cm; branch bark smooth, gray; leaves leathery, with 10-20 leaflets, each 5-10 cm long; flowers in large panicles, white, 4-6 mm long; fruit a drupe, 1.5-2 cm long, red, turning black when ripe, with thick white pulp.

Habitat: Forests, roadsides.

Traditional Uses: Bark and root yield a powerful astringent used for *dysentery, diarrhea, hemorrhage, excessive menstruation,* and *internal bleeding.* As a *tonic,* especially for stomach and bowels, boil a small handful of chopped bark in 3 cups water for 10 minutes and use as tea or bath. Boil bark or root to wash *sores.*

The wood is used for house frames and broomsticks.

Research Results: *Simarouba glauca* var. *latifolia* has shown activity against malaria in studies in chickens. A water extract was used at a dose of 10 mg/kg, and a chloroform extract was used at a dose of 1.0 mg/kg against *Plasmodium gallinaceum*; both showed strong activity (Spencer et al. 1947). The plant is known to contain triterpenes and lipids. The active principles are mixtures of degraded triterpenes (quassinoids, simaroubolides) (Farnsworth 1993).

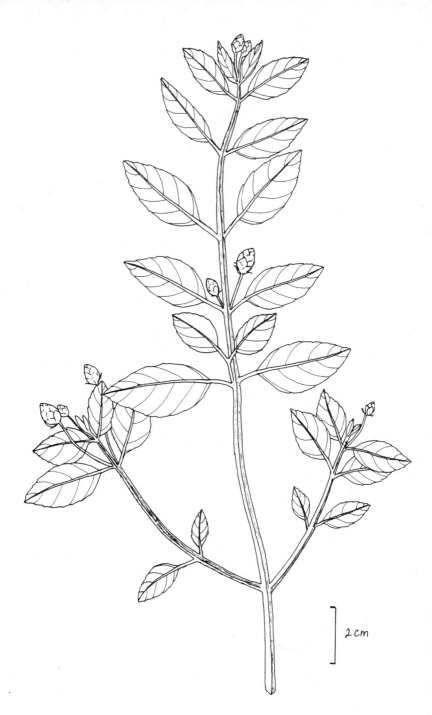

Lippia dulcis Trev.

122

ORASÚS (S)

Scientific Name: *Lippia dulcis* Trev.

Plant Family: Verbenaceae

Description: Small runner herb to 20 cms; leaves dark green, 1-6 cm long, with strong scent and sweet flavor; flower spikes to 3 cm long, with flowers 1-1.5 mm long; seeds black.

Habitat: Pastures, yards, clearings, moist thickets, ponds.

Traditional Uses: A favorite remedy for *bronchitis* and *dry, hacking coughs* -- boil a handful of fresh plant material with 1 cup of sugar in 1 quart water for 10 minutes; allow steam from boiled herbs to penetrate chest area by wrapping a towel around patient with steaming pot in front of chest. Strain off after steaming has stopped and drink hot in sips all day until the mucus comes out. Chew flowers for *toothache*; apply over tooth on gum. The leaves are intensely sweet.

Research Results: A tincture of dried flowers, leaf, and stem was shown to have expectorant activity in humans and showed clinical improvement in 5 of 10 patients treated for bronchitis (Compadre and Kinghorn 1985). Classes of chemicals in this plant include monoterpenes, sesquiterpenes, alkenes (ibid.), and vitamins (Compadre et al. 1986).

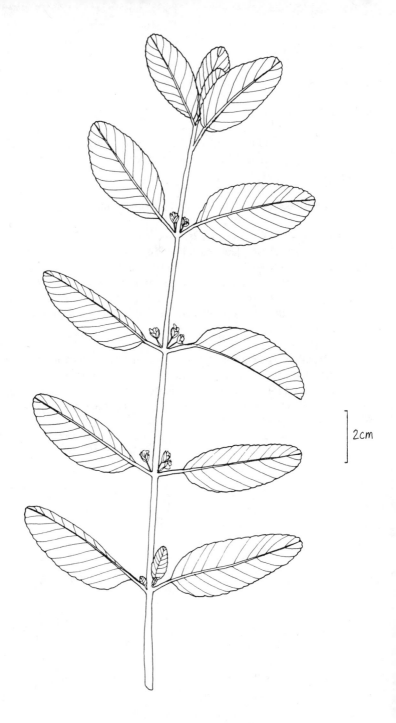

Lippia graveolens HBK.

OREGANO

Scientific Name: *Lippia graveolens* HBK.

Plant Family: Verbenaceae

Description: A shrub to 2 m tall; stems woody; leaves green, obovate, to 4-5 cm long x 1-3 cm wide, aromatic; flowers appearing in axils of leaves, white, ca. 5 mm long.

Habitat: Commonly cultivated, and escaped in yards and gardens.

Traditional Uses: Known as both food and medicine to all cultures in Belize. Fresh and dried leaves are added to soups, stews, and sauces, imparting flavor and aiding digestion.

Highly respected as a medicinal plant, it is used as a tea for *upper respiratory tract infections*, and to induce *menstruation* or *increase a scanty flow*. For tea, pour 3 cups of boiling water over 1/2 cup of freshly picked leaves (or 3 tablespoons dried leaves) and allow to steep for 15 minutes; strain and drink 1 cup of hot tea before each meal as needed. Drink 1 glass of warm decoction of leaves for 7 days after childbirth to *clean uterus*. To make an excellent wash for *wounds, infections*, and *burns* (especially if septic), boil 1 quart of fresh leaves (or a handful of dried leaves) in 1 gallon of water for 10 minutes; when cooled, wash affected areas 3 times daily and allow treated areas to air dry.

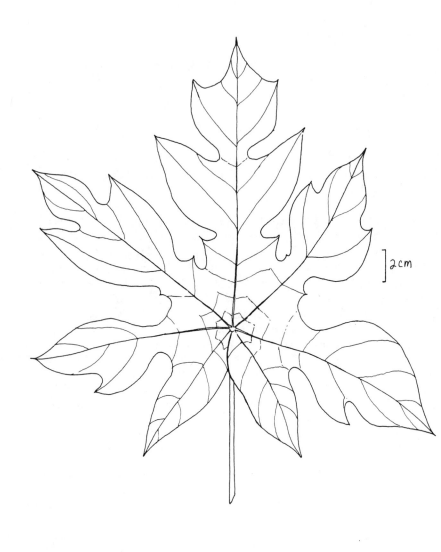

]2cm

Carica papaya L.

PAPAYA

Scientific Name: *Carica papaya* L.

Plant Family: Caricaceae

Description: Shrub or small tree with thick trunk growing to 3-6 m tall; leaves large, palmately-lobed, green, growing along the upper half of stem, or along the upper quarter in older plants; flowers white, with separate staminate and pistillate plants; fruits obovoid to oblong, hanging from the stem; copious latex contained in the stems, leaves, and fruit.

Habitat: A cultivated plant, but wild forms also found at edge of disturbed forest, old fields, roadsides.

Traditional Uses: Fruits are sweet and edible; especially nice as a juice. If taken in excess, will act as a *purge*. Slice fruit, crush seeds, and apply to *wounds, cuts*, and *infections* to aid healing. To reduce redness and promote healing of irritation from fire coral, rub very ripe (even rotting) fruit into affected area. Wrap raw meat in leaves to tenderize; it will be ready to remove after 1-2 hours. Slice stem and gather juice; apply to *corns* on feet to dissolve. Slice green fruits and gather milky sap -- apply to *warts*. Ripe flesh of fruit is eaten for *constipation, sluggish liver,* as a *diuretic,* for *indigestion,* and for *high blood pressure.* Boiled root is used in a formula for *venereal disease.*

Research Results: Papaya is a widely studied plant from the pharmacological perspective. Hundreds of individual tests appear in the literature, noting both activity and inactivity in a variety of screens. The active results include: *in vitro* antibacterial activity from fresh epicarp tissue against *Bacillus cereus, Pseudomonas aeruginosa, Shigella flexneri*, and *Staphylococcus aureus* (Emeruwa 1982); cardiac depressent activity in humans from a hot water extract of the fruit at 0.2 gm/person (Noble 1947); ascaricidal activity in dogs from a 1.50 ml/kg dose, effective against *Ascaris lumbricoides* (Nagaty et al. 1959); antiyeast activity (*Candida albicans*) from a 10% concentration of latex *in vitro*, with similar results against *Candida guillierinondii* and *Candida tropicalis* (Tezuka and Kitabatake 1980); and *in vitro* antifungal activity from an ethanol extract of the fresh leaf (10% concentration) against *Neurospora crassa* (Rojas Hernández et al. 1981).

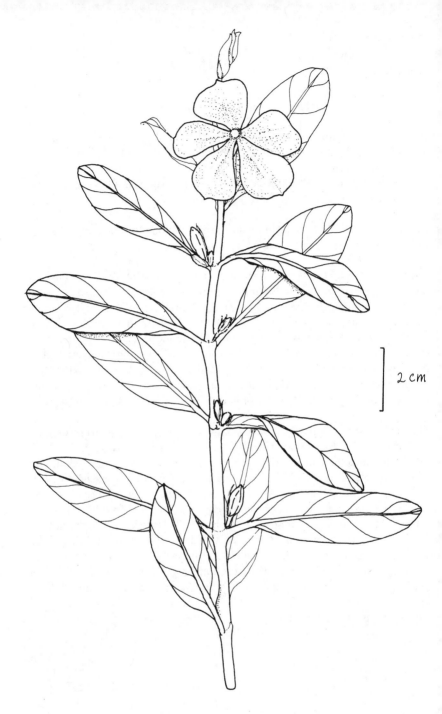

Catharanthus roseus (L.) G. Don

PERIWINKLE

Ram Goat (E)
Chata, Picaria (S)
All Day Flower (Men.)

Scientific Name: *Catharanthus roseus* (L.) G. Don

Plant Family: Apocynaceae

Description: Common wild and semi-cultivated herb growing to 1 m; leaves shiny, bright green; flowers pink, 2 cm across, borne at ends of stems.

Habitat: Cultivated, and naturalized in roadsides and old fields.

Traditional Uses: The leafy stems are used as a tea for *diabetes, menopause, high blood pressure*, and to slow the growth of *tumors* -- boil two 30 cm long branches in 3 cups of water for 2 minutes; steep for 15 minutes; strain and drink 3 cups daily before meals. Soak 9 pink flowers in one pint of water for 3 hours in sunlight and take sips all day for *sore throat* and *colds*.

Research Results: This is an extremely well-studied plant that is the source of two potent cancer-fighting alkaloids, vincristine and vinblastine. The plant, originally under study for its folk use to treat diabetes, was found to contain alkaloids that are now crucial in the battle against Hodgkins' disease and childhood leukemia. Seventy-two alkaloids have been isolated from this plant. Approximately 500 kg of whole plant is required to make a single gram of the alkaloid. Interestingly, its effectiveness in the treatment of diabetes is not verified by laboratory research on animal models. Westbrooks and Preacher (1986) note that excessive consumption or long-term use of this plant may cause kidney and nervous system disorders.

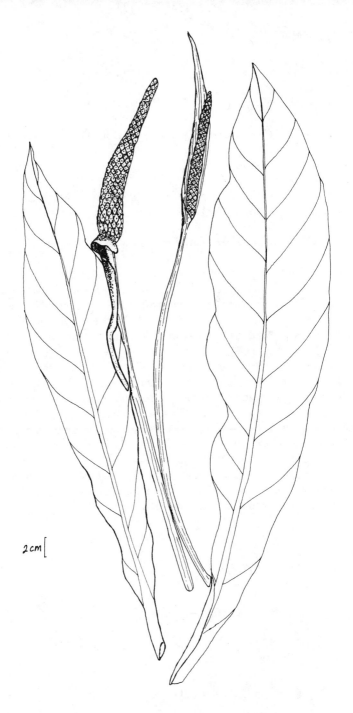

2 cm [

Anthurium schlechtendalii Kunth.

PHEASANT TAIL

Cola de Faisán (S)
Xiv-yak-tun-ich (M)

Scientific Name: *Anthurium schlechtendalii* Kunth.

Plant Family: Araceae

Description: Large herbaceous plant; leaves dark green, leathery, to 1 m long, arising from a cluster of white cordlike roots; flowers with a dark purple bract, borne on tall spike to 70 cm long; fruits, when ripe, are small red berries to 1 cm in diameter.

Habitat: Wet forests, rocky hillsides or outcrops, on trees.

Traditional Uses: The leaves are used to treat *sprains, aches, rheumatism, arthritis, paralysis, backaches, muscle spasms* -- boil 3 large leaves in 2 gallons water for 10 minutes. Use this mixture when warm to bathe *painful muscles, joints,* or *sprains.* For *severe cramps, spasms,* or *paralysis,* use only steam from boiling leaves; place limb or affected area over the steam coming from the boiling leaves and cover with blanket, being careful not to burn skin. For *backache* or *muscle spasm,* mash center vein of leaf and apply leaf to painful area; place hot water bottle over this for one hour -- this technique can be very helpful. Also, a poultice of mashed leaf is applied to the skin for *pain* and *swelling* -- it will stick to the affected part and can be worn all day.

Research Results: No information was located on the bioactivity of this species. However, an ethanol extract of the flowers of *Anthurium andraeanum* was shown to have *in vitro* activity against *Staphylococcus aureus* (Avirutnant and Pongpan 1983).

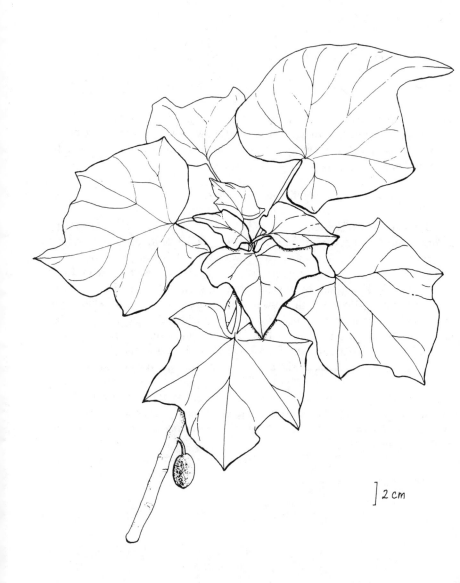

Jatropha curcas L.

PHYSIC NUT

Scientific Name: *Jatropha curcas* L.

Plant Family: Euphorbiaceae

Description: Shrub growing to 2 m, with spreading branches; leaves have clear sap when broken from stem; flowers white; seed capsules ellipsoidal, 2.5-4 cm long.

Habitat: Semi-cultivated in fields and clearings.

Traditional Uses: The clear sap which runs from the stem and ends of leaves is gathered and used to treat *mouth sores* and *infantile thrush* by rubbing sap directly on membrane of mouth. Leaves are boiled (1 leaf per cup of water for 5 minutes) to make a mouthwash for conditions of the *gums* and *throat*, and drunk as a tea for *stoppage of urine, constipation, burning inside body, backache*, and *inflammation of ovaries*. Dried seeds are ground and boiled to use as a strong *purgative*, but these can be quite toxic if not properly prepared (see below).

Boil a 7.5 cm x 7.5 cm strip of bark together with 6 leaves in 1/2 quart of water for 5 minutes to use as a douche for *vaginitis*. For *spleen* complaints, boil 9 cut up young limes with 3 leaves for 10 minutes in 1/2 gallon of water and drink daily in place of water.

Research Results: This species is in the same family as the castor bean and the oil also serves as a purgative. Kingsbury (1964) reports that there are many incidents of poisonings in humans from overdoses of the oil and consumption of the seed. He notes that there appears to be a difference between plants in the toxicity of their seeds; in some cases, only 3 seeds have caused toxicity. Thus, caution is advised when using the plant. The TRAMIL 4 workshop advised against any internal use of this plant, due to its toxicity (Robineau 1991).

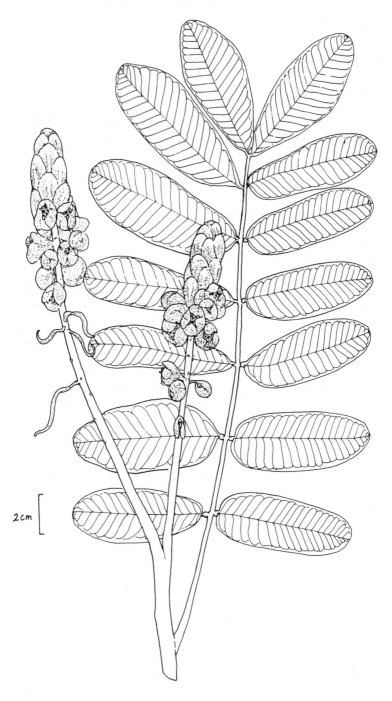

Senna alata (L.) Roxb.

134

PISS A BED (C)

Shrimp Flower (E)
Hoja de Barajas (S)

Scientific Name: *Senna alata* (L.) Roxb.

Plant Family: Caesalpiniaceae

Description: Shrub growing to 2 m tall, with many branches; leaves consist of 6-12 pairs of leaflets; yellow flowers borne in racemes at the ends or in the axils of the leaves.

Habitat: Yards and patios; also in disturbed forests.

Traditional Uses: Named for its history as an excellent remedy for *urinary tract* conditions. For this purpose, 3 bunches of flowers are boiled in 3 cups water for 2 minutes and steeped for 15 minutes; drink 3 cups in sips all day. Boil the leaves as a remedy for *liver congestion, liver spots, kidney ailments,* and as a purge for the *lymph system.* Use fresh leaf juice for *ringworm* and *scabies.* Standley and Steyermark (1946) note that the popular English name of the plant in Guatemala is "ringworm shrub," due to its use as a remedy in tropical America for this and other skin diseases. For *female infertility,* soak 8 ounces of mashed roots in 1 quart of anise liquor for 5 days; take 1 ounce of this tincture daily for 10 days before onset of menstruation.

Research Results: Anti-inflammatory activity in rats has been shown from an ethanol-water (1:1) extract of the fresh plant at a dose of 500 mg/kg (Dhawan et al. 1977). *In vitro* antibacterial activity against *Escherichia coli, Klebsiella pneumoniae, Serratia marcescens,* and *Staphylococcus aureus* resulted from a 95% ethanol extract (Benjamin 1980). *In vitro* antifungal activity against *Trichophyton mentagrophytes* was shown from a hot water extract of dried leaf at a 5% concentration (Fuzellier et al. 1982).

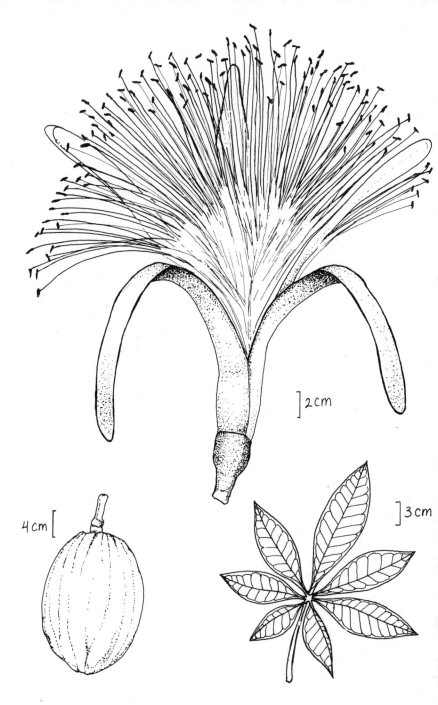

2cm

4cm

3cm

Pachira aquatica Aubl.

PROVISION BARK

Santo Domingo, Bobo (S)
Cuyche (M)

Scientific Name: *Pachira aquatica* Aubl.

Plant Family: Bombacaceae

Description: A tree growing to 10-20 m tall; trunk buttressed, to 60 cm in diameter; bark light brown or gray, smooth; leaves with 5-8 leathery leaflets, each 8-20 cm long; flowers white, petals 18-30 cm long, with long purple stamens; fruit ovoid to 20-30 cm long, light brown.

Habitat: Along rivers and streams; in forests and fields.

Traditional Uses: A popular beverage tea to *build the blood* in old age, to treat *anemia* and *exhaustion*, and for *low blood pressure.* For *kidney pain*, cut a seed from the fruit in quarters; boil in 1 cup of water for 5 minutes and drink before breakfast for 3 consecutive days. Boil a piece of bark 2.5 x 10 cm in 3 cups water for 10 minutes; drink 1/2 cup 6 times daily as a general tonic to *build blood and strength*. Standley and Steyermark (1949) report that the seeds are cooked and eaten in some parts of Central America.

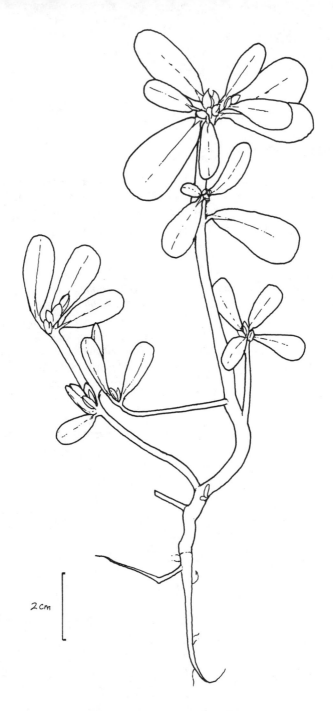

2 cm

Portulaca oleracea L.

PURSLANE

Verdolaga (S)
Xucul (M)

Scientific Name: *Portulaca oleracea* L.

Plant Family: Portulacaceae

Description: A fleshy annual plant that creeps along the ground and grows to 20-40 cm long; stems shiny; leaves shiny, 1-3 cm long, fleshy; flowers yellow, clustered at tips of the stems; seeds black, round, 1 mm in diameter.

Habitat: Old fields, yards, gardens, damp places.

Traditional Uses: The leaves and stems of the plant are useful as a *diuretic*, to *clean the blood*, and to *nourish the system* (especially for convalescents), as they are rich in minerals, protein, and Vitamin C -- boil 1 large plant in 3 cups water for 5 minutes. Crush the fresh plant material to apply as a poultice to stop *bleeding* and heal *ulcers, wounds,* and *sores*. Fresh juice of the plant can be taken with sugar and honey to relieve *dry coughs*. Mash stems and leaves to apply as a poultice over the forehead to alleviate *headaches* caused by over-exposure to the sun. Said to be a cooling plant. This plant is both medicine and food. Boil the leaves and stems in a bit of water for 10 minutes; add salt, oil, seasonings and serve. Add it raw to salads. The thick, older stems can be pickled in salt and vinegar.

Research Results: A dose of 1.5 and 2.0 gm/kg of the entire dried plant showed hypoglycemic activity in rabbits after 8 and 12 hours (Akhtar et al. 1985). Uterine stimulant effect was demonstrated in mice and rats using a water extract of the leaves (Sharaf 1969). *In vitro* antibacterial activity was shown using an acetone extract of dried leaves in *Pseudomonas aeruginosa*; an ethanol (95%) extract with *Escherichia coli, Pseudomonas aeruginosa, Salmonella typhosa, Sarcina lutea, Serratia marcescens, Shigella flexneri, Staphylococcus albus, Staphylococcus aureus*; and a water extract with *Escherichia coli, Pseudomonas aeruginosa,* and *Serratia marcescens* (Jiménez Misas et al. 1979a). Smooth muscle relaxant activity was obtained using an ethanol (95%) extract of leaf and stem at a concentration of 0.33 ml/1 in rabbits, and a water extract at a concentration of 0.33 ml/l in rabbits (Feng et al. 1962). It should be noted that this plant is a source of omega-3 fatty acids, such as found in fish, and thus is a vegetable "substitute" for fish oil (Simopoulos and Salem 1987). It is also a good source of antioxidants such as alpha-tocopherol, ascorbic acid, beta-carotene, and glutathione (Simopoulos et al. 1992).

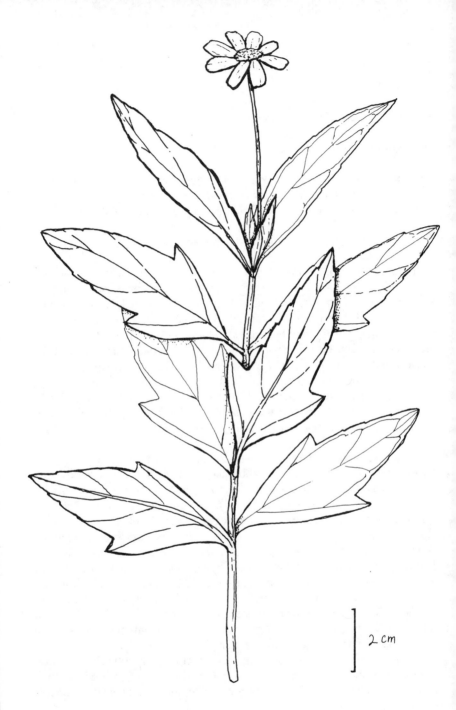

Wedelia trilobata (L.) Hitchc.

RABBIT'S PAW

Pasmo (M)
Dungya (Garífuna)

Scientific Name: *Wedelia trilobata* (L.) Hitchc.

Plant Family: Asteraceae

Description: Low growing or creeping herbaceous perennial, 50 cm-1 m long; leaves 3-12 cm long, often with 3 lobes; flowers solitary, yellow, ca. 2-3 cm across.

Habitat: Clearings, roadsides, fields, gardens.

Traditional Uses: Used for *hepatitis, indigestion* due to sluggish liver, *white stools, burning in the urine* and *stoppage of urine,* and for *infections* -- boil 1 cup of fresh herb (stems, leaves, and flowers) in 3 cups water for 5 minutes and drink 1 cup warm before each meal. To bathe those suffering from *backache, muscle cramps, rheumatism,* or *swellings,* boil a large double handful of fresh stems and leaves in 2 gallons of water for 10 minutes. Said to pull "heat" out of the body. For painful joints of *arthritis,* mash fresh leaves and stems; spread on a cloth and apply to area, wrapping securely with a warm covering.

Research Results: *Wedelia trilobata* contains sesquiterpenes, diterpenes, alkenynes, sulfur compounds (Bohlmann and Ngo-Le-Van 1977); triterpenes (Bohlmann et al. 1981), and monoterpenes (Mancini 1980).

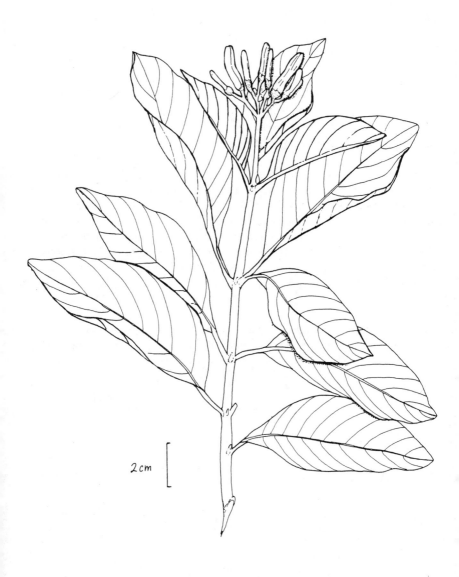

Hamelia patens Jacq.

RED HEAD

Polly Red Head (E)
Sanalo-todo (S)
Ix-canan (M)

Scientific Name: *Hamelia patens* Jacq.

Plant Family: Rubiaceae

Description: Semi-woody shrub to 3 m tall; leaves deeply veined, red-tinted, to 6-20 cm long; flowers bright orange-red, tubular; fruit a red berry, turning black when ripe.

Habitat: Pastures, old fields, roadsides.

Traditional Uses: Ix-canan, meaning "guardian of the forest" in Maya, is used to treat all *skin problems, sores, rashes, burns, itching, cuts, fungus*, and *insect bites* -- boil a large double handful of flowers, leaves, and stems in 2 gallons of water for 10 minutes; bathe area with warm mixture. Dry and powder plant to sprinkle on stubborn sores or ulcers after bathing with plant parts as above; cover with gauze and keep clean. Make decoction from entire plant and use as sitz bath or drink as tea (3 cups daily) to alleviate *menstrual cramps/pain*. For *sting* from bees, wasps or "doctor fly," apply warmed leaf as poultice or crush fresh leaves and rub juice on sting. The fruits are edible.

To make a household "iodine," boil 3 stems approximately 25 cm long in 3 cups of water for 10 minutes; add rusty nail for 15 minutes; strain off and bottle.

Research Results: Tests with this plant show a great deal of biological activity, especially in the antibacterial and antifungal area. For example, an ethanol (95%) extract of dried leaf yielded *in vitro* activity against *Staphylococcus aureus*, and a water extract was active against *Escherichia coli, Salmonella typhosa, Sarcina lutea, Serratia marcescens*, and *Shigella flexneri* (Jiménez Misas et al. 1979b). Analgesic activity was shown in rats from a methanol extract of dried leaf at a dose of 770 mg/kg (Esposito-Avella 1985). Antifungal activity against *Neurospora crassa* was shown in ethanol, acetone, and water extracts of dried stem at a concentration of 50% (López Abraham et al. 1981).

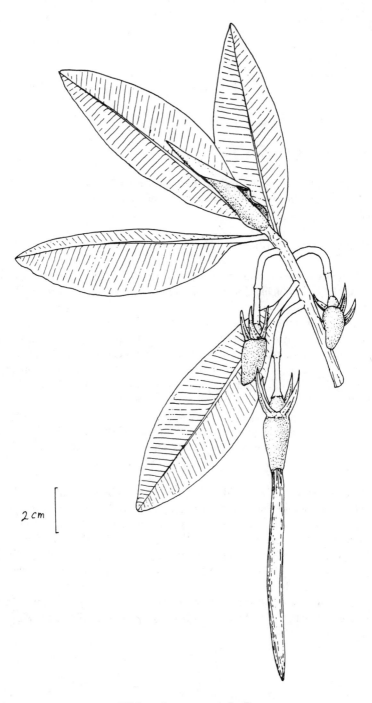

2 cm

Rhizophora mangle L.

RED MANGROVE

Mangle, Mangle Colorado (S)

Scientific Name: *Rhizophora mangle* L.

Plant Family: Rhizophoraceae

Description: Tree or shrub to 10-25 m tall, often with many stilt roots; stem diameter less than 1 m; leaves leathery, 5-15 cm long by ca. 3 cm wide, dark green above, light green on underside; flowers yellow, ca. 1 cm long; fruits 10-15 cm long.

Habitat: Growing in forests along the sea or inland in salty, swampy areas.

Traditional Uses: The bark of the tree is boiled (1 handful of chopped bark in 1 gallon of water for 10 minutes) and used as a hot bath for very stubborn or serious *sores, skin conditions, leprosy,* and *swellings.*

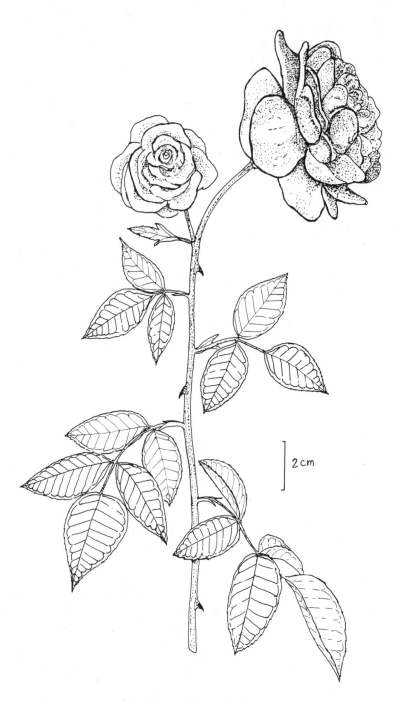

Rosa chinensis Jacq.

RED ROSE

Rosa (S)

Scientific Name: *Rosa chinensis* Jacq.

Plant Family: Rosaceae

Description: Shrub to 2 m tall; stems shiny, thorny; leaves 2-3 cm long; flowers red, 10 cm in diameter, fragrant.

Habitat: Cultivated in yards, patios, gardens.

Traditional Uses: A "cooling" plant for *fevers*, and binding or astringent for *infantile* or *childhood diarrhea* -- steep 1 red rose and 9 leaves in 1 cup boiling water for 15 minutes; strain and drink. Use same infusion as a *tonic* cordial. A stronger infusion using 3 red roses and a handful of leaves steeped for 15 minutes in 1 cup hot water is useful against *adult diarrhea* and *hemorrhage*. All infusions should be allowed to cool before drinking.

Research Results: A methanol extract of the flowers showed *in vitro* antifungal activity against *Alternaria humicola, Alternaria solani, Cephalosporium sacchari, Curvularia lunata, Curvularia pallescens, Fusarium nivale, Fusarium oxysporum, Helminthosporium oryzae, Helminthosporium sativum, Pythium aphanidermatum*, and *Rhizopus nigricans* (Tripathi and Dixit 1977). Avirutnant and Pongpan (1983) report the following laboratory results: *in vitro* antibacterial activity against *Salmonella typhosa, Shigella dysenteriae*, and *Staphylococcus aureus* from both an ethanol (95%) extract of dried flowers at a concentration of 100 mg/disc and a water extract at a concentration of 20 mg/disc; antiyeast activity against *Candida albicans* in both an ethanol (95%) extract at a concentration of 100 mg/disc and a water extract at a concentration of 20 mg/disc.

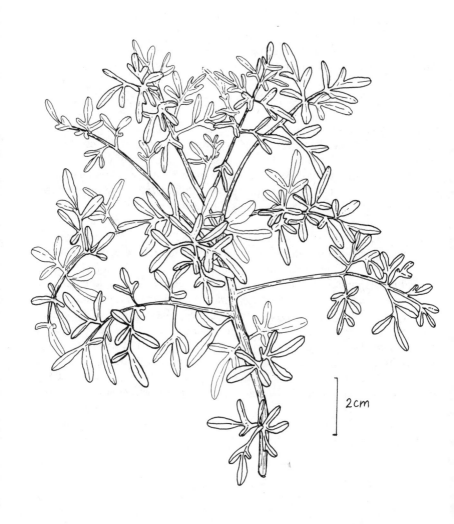

2cm

Ruta graveolens L.

RUE

Ruda (S)
Sink-in (M)

Scientific Name: *Ruta graveolens* L.

Plant Family: Rutaceae

Description: A glaucous shrubby herb to 1 m tall; leaves to 1 cm long, with a strong odor; flowers yellow.

Habitat: Escaped cultivation in places, but mostly a yard pot plant found in many homes throughout Belize.

Traditional Uses: Rue is seldom boiled; generally 9 small branches are squeezed into a glass of water, strained and drunk twice daily before meals for *stomach cramps, late menses,* to kill *intestinal worms,* to prevent attacks of *epilepsy,* to stop *vomiting,* and *to calm the nerves.* To ease *childbirth* and *aid contractions,* sip rue water during delivery. Soak rue leaves in alcohol to use as a linament on *sore muscles, backache, headache, muscle spasms,* and to massage those suffering from *fever, exhaustion,* or *fainting spells.*

Rue has a reputation as a useful plant against all *spiritual diseases* such as witchcraft, envy, evil eye, fright, and grief. Sufferers may eat the fresh leaves, or prepare a drink or bath with them.

Research Results: Numerous studies have been carried out on this plant, which is commonly cultivated in many parts of the world. It has abortifacient activity with intoxication manifested by vomiting, salivation, epigastric pain, delerium, tremors, and collapse with a slow irregular pulse. NAPRALERT notes that it is "frequently fatal for mother" (Papavassiliou and Eliakis 1937). When used as an insect repellent (rubbed on the skin), it produces phyto-photodermatitis with symptoms of erythema, hyperpigmentation, and blistering (Heskel et al. 1983). There are many other reports of similar results when using this plant on the skin. Caution is advised. An ethanol (95%) extract was shown to have anticonvulsant activity in mice at a dose of 2-4 ml/kg (Athanassova-Shopova et al. 1965). Both antibacterial activity against *Bacillus subtilis* and anti-tuberculosis activity against *Mycobacterium phlei* were obtained using ethanol (95%) extracts of dried root on an agar plate (Nahrstedt et al. 1981).

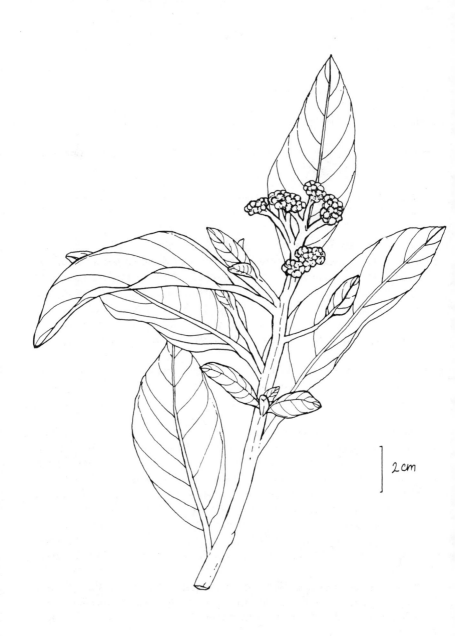

] 2 cm

Croton guatemalensis Lotsy

SANTA MARIA (S)

Pito Sico (S)
Chal-che (M)

Scientific Name: *Croton guatemalensis* Lotsy

Plant Family: Euphorbiaceae

Description: Shrub growing to 3 m, with many branches; leaves rough to the touch with an aroma reminiscent of oregano; flowers borne in clusters at tips of branches, pale orange, turning brown.

Habitat: Clearings, roadsides, at edge of forested areas.

Traditional Uses: Leaves are boiled to make steam bath for mothers after *childbirth* to insure that there is no infection and that reproductive organs return to their proper position -- a large double handful of leaves is boiled in about 2 gallons of water for 15 minutes and the woman is made to sit over steaming pot for 30 minutes. Leaves are also used to make a tea which is drunk *after childbirth* to assist healing and for difficult *menstruation* and *uterine problems* -- a small handful of leaves is boiled for 5 minutes in 3 cups of water. For *painful joints*, heat fresh leaves in oil and apply directly to the area affected.

This is the "male" Chal-che; the female is the following entry, *Pluchea symphytifolia*. Their common names in Spanish are identical.

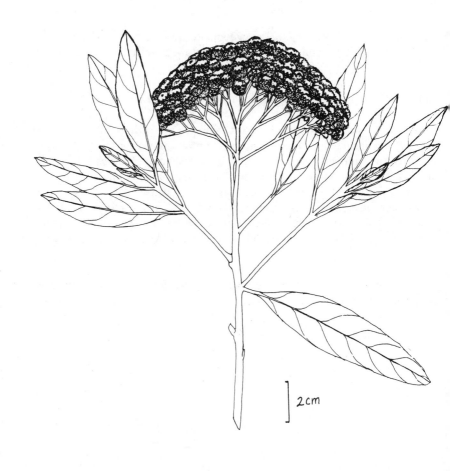

] 2cm

Pluchea symphytifolia (Mill.) Gillis

SANTA MARIA (S)

Pito Sico (S)
Ix Chal-che (M)

Scientific Name: *Pluchea symphytifolia* (Mill.) Gillis

Plant Family: Asteraceae

Description: Woody shrub to 3 m tall with many branches; leaves aromatic, to 7-15 cm long; flowers brownish green in large heads, turning orange.

Habitat: Clearings, old fields, edge of forests.

Traditional Uses: Boil 3 leaves in 3 cups water for 2 minutes; steep for 15 minutes and drink 3 cups very hot over 3 hour period for onset of *asthma attacks*, or take slowly all day for *coughs, colds,* and *flu*. After *childbirth*, boil a large double handful of leaves in 1 gallon of water for 10 minutes; woman sits over steaming pot of herbs for 20 minutes with towel wrapped around her and pot to allow steam to be absorbed into vagina -- this will insure that uterus returns to proper position and will prevent infection and excessive bleeding. Also used to bathe *swellings, tumors, inflammations,* and *bruises*. Warm a few leaves in oil; wrap these in a piece of cotton or flannel and apply as a poultice over *sore muscles, rheumatic pains, neuritis,* and *arthritic joints*.

This is the "female" Chal-che; the male is *Croton guatemalensis* (preceding page). Their common names in Spanish are identical.

Research Results: This plant, noted in the pharmacological literature as *Pluchea odorata*, has shown antifungal activity against *Neurospora crassa*. An ethanol (95%) extract of dried leaf was used in agar plate at a concentration of 50% (López Abraham et al. 1981). Ethanol and acetone extracts of dried stem showed antifungal activity against *Neurospora crassa in vitro* at a concentration of 50% (ibid.). Insecticidal activity was obtained from a methanol extract of dried shoots at 5 mg concentration against *Anostrepa ludens* (Domínguez S. and Alcorn 1985).

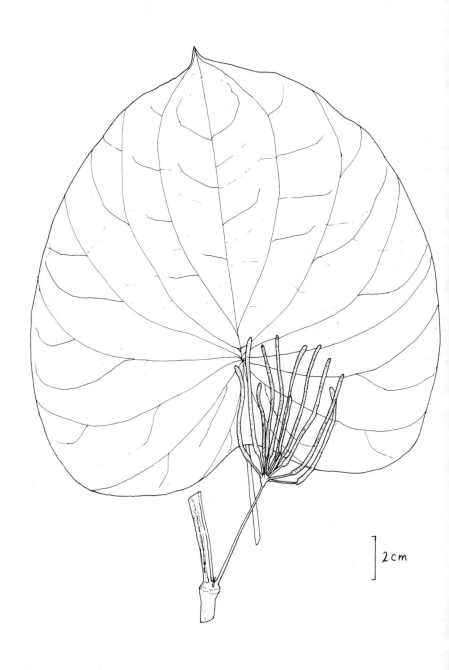

Pothomorphe peltata (L.) Miq.

154

SANTIAGO (S)

San Diego (S)
U-tu-it (M)

Scientific Name: *Pothomorphe peltata* (L.) Miq.

Plant Family: Piperaceae

Description: Large herb growing to 2 m tall, with few branches; leaves heart-shaped, highly aromatic, large, to 20-30 cm long; inflorescence a white or pale green spike, 8-9 cm long x 3.5 mm thick and occurring in groups of 4-10.

Habitat: Roadsides and rocky outcroppings.

Traditional Uses: This leaf is highly respected for its ability to alleviate the pain of *muscle spasm, headache,* and *stomachache* -- warm a large leaf and apply to painful area; cover with a towel and rest. For *backache,* heat a large leaf in small amount of cooking oil and apply to painful area overnight; cover with towels and keep warm. Also useful as an herbal bath for *rheumatism* and *arthritis.* Used to *stimulate milk production* in women -- bathe back and breasts with a warm tea of the leaf.

Research Results: Little information is available on the chemistry or biological activity of this plant. Dried leaf is reportedly used as an antifertility agent in both Brazil and Ecuador (González and Silva 1987).

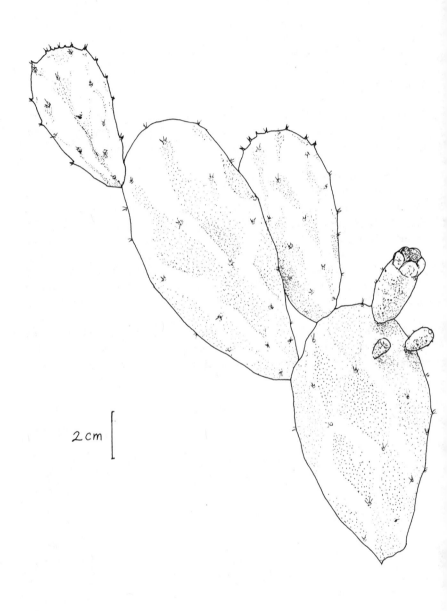

2cm

Opuntia ficus-indica (L.) Mill.

SCOGGINEAL (C)

Nopal, Tuna (S)

Scientific Name: *Opuntia ficus-indica* (L.) Mill.

Plant Family: Cactaceae

Description: A cactus growing to 3 m tall, with large thorny pads (sometimes referred to as "leaves") to 40 cm or longer; flowers red; fruits red-pink.

Habitat: Old fields, yards, doorsteps.

Traditional Uses: Peel, slice, and tie fresh pad around head to relieve *headaches* and *fever*. Boil 1 pad in 3 cups water for 5 minutes; drink 1 cup before each meal for *high blood pressure, fever*, and *malaise*. Crush and soak 5 fresh pads in 1 gallon water -- use as rinse to *prevent falling hair*; drink as tea for *bladder conditions*. Drink 1 cup of juice from fresh pad at onset of *childbirth* to ease delivery. Midwives also recommend ingesting 1/4 cup daily for 7-10 days prior to delivery. Eat peeled, steamed, and chilled pads in salad to alleviate *arthritis*. The fruit is edible and highly esteemed -- the spiny, outer portion is peeled off, and the red or yellowish seedy center is consumed (it has a crunchy, sweet taste). Caution must be taken to avoid eating the small hair-like spines (called glochids) found on the outside of the fruit.

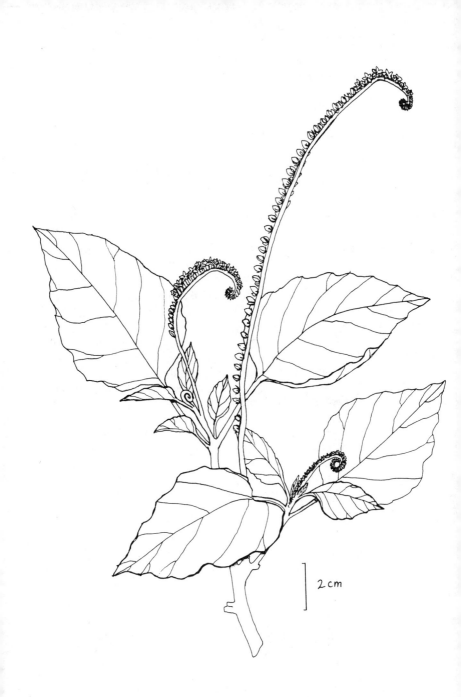

Heliotropium indicum L.

SCORPION'S TAIL

Rabomico, Cola de Alacrán (S)

Scientific Name: *Heliotropium indicum* L.

Plant Family: Boraginaceae

Description: Upright annual herb growing to 1 m tall; leaves green, rough in texture; flowers small, white, borne on end of curled stem that resembles a scorpion's tail.

Habitat: Old fields, clearings, yards.

Traditional Uses: For *diarrhea, malaise* or *vomiting* in infants -- boil an entire plant in 1 gallon water for 5 minutes and bathe infant in warm water at bedtime. Use tea bath for *skin conditions*. Take unsweetened tea for *painful periods* or *scanty flow*. To prepare tea, boil 3 15-cm long stem pieces with leaves for 5 minutes in 3 cups water and drink warm. Note that the plant can be *toxic* if drunk regularly or in large doses. Boil 3 leaves in 1 cup water for 10 minutes and strain through cloth to use as *eye wash*.

Research Results: A substantial amount of phytochemical screening has been carried out on this plant. Numerous pyrrolizidine alkaloids are present in the plant. Biological activities reported include uterine stimulant effect in rats from a water extract of roots (Barros et al. 1970); uterine stimulant effect in rats from an ethanol extract of roots (Vieira et al. 1968); antispasmodic activity of an unspecified type from a dried seed extract. in guinea pigs (Pandey et al. 1982). Long-term medicinal use of this plant could result in liver damage and/or cancer due to the presence of pyrrolizidine alkaloids (Farnsworth 1993).

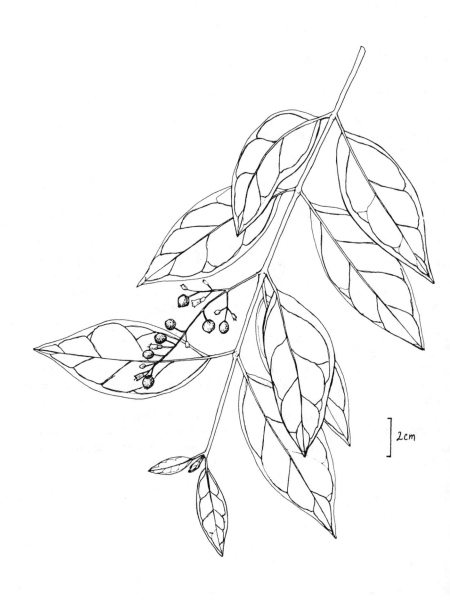

Chiococca alba (L.) Hitchc.

SKUNK ROOT

Zorillo (S)
Pay-che (M)

Scientific Name: *Chiococca alba* (L.) Hitchc.

Plant Family: Rubiaceae

Description: A vining shrub to 3 m tall; stem is somewhat square in shape and when cut or peeled has a strong odor reminiscent of a skunk; flowers white; fruits white, 4-8 mm long; seeds dark brown, 3-4 mm long.

Habitat: Forests, especially on hillsides.

Traditional Uses: The action of zorillo on the body is very strong -- care must be taken when using this remedy as it often proves to be too potent for the elderly and the very weak. For *delayed menstruation, ulcers* of the stomach or intestines, *constipation, obstructed bowels, colitis, endometriosis, pain, nervousness, dementia*, and *depression*, boil a small handful of chopped root in 3 cups of water for 10 minutes; strain and drink 1 cup before each meal. Children should take 1 cup daily in sips throughout the day for any of the above ailments.

Prepare as above and use as an excellent skin wash for *stubborn sores, rashes*, and *ulcers*. For *alcoholism*, place one handful of chopped root in about 1 quart of rum, vodka, or gin. Soak in sun for five days and strain. Persons wishing to kick the habit must take one shot daily of this mixture or be allowed to finish the entire quart at once. They will vomit violently, after which it is said that the smell of alcohol will make them nauseous for years to come.

Used to dispel *witchcraft* and *evil eye*, and drunk by shamans to strengthen *spiritual powers*. Said to be the "thinking herb" of the Maya -- able to give relief in a great variety of complaints and used when all else fails or the practitioner is unsure of the ailment.

Research Results: An ethanol extract of the dried leaf of zorillo showed *in vitro* cytotoxic activity (KB cancer cell line -- 65% inhibition of cell growth) as did similar extracts of the stem (77.5% inhibition of cell growth) and root (69.6% inhibition of cell growth) (Nascimento et al. 1990). Compounds identified in zorillo include coumarins, alkanes, carbohydrates, and lignans (El-Hafiz et al. 1991).

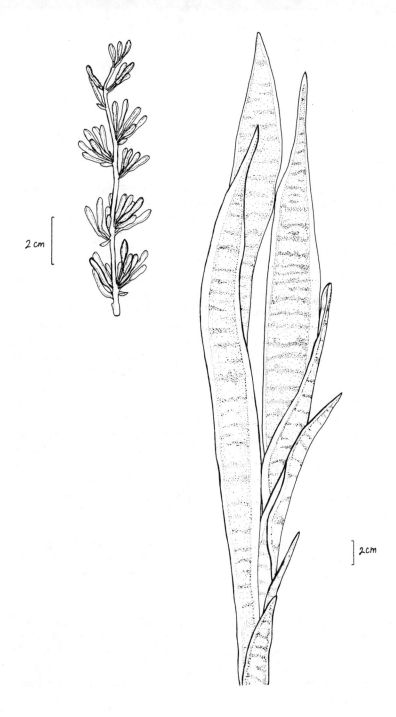

2 cm

2 cm

Sansevieria trifasciata Prain.

SNAKE PLANT

Culebrilla, Lengua de Vaca (S)

Scientific Name: *Sansevieria trifasciata* Prain.

Plant Family: Agavaceae

Description: A stemless plant; leaves stiff, thick, erect, to 50 cm long x 4 cm wide, colored with light green and dark green cross bands; flowers greenish white, to 1 cm long, clustered on a raceme to ca. 75 cm long.

Habitat: Gardens, yards, edge of forests, old fields, escaped from cultivation.

Traditional Uses: Boil the leaves to bathe skin *sores* and *rashes*. Mash leaves and put extracted juice into chicken water to prevent *diseases of fowl* in the barnyard. The fresh leaves are chewed for *snakebite* and *diabetes*. A fiber is extracted from the pounded leaves to make rope.

Research Results: According to the pharmacological literature, this plant has been evaluated against a number of screens, most of which showed no activity. Der Marderosian et al. (1976) found toxicity in the flowers in studies of rats and mice using a water extract at an unspecified dose. The plant is known to contain saponins and glycosides (ibid.).

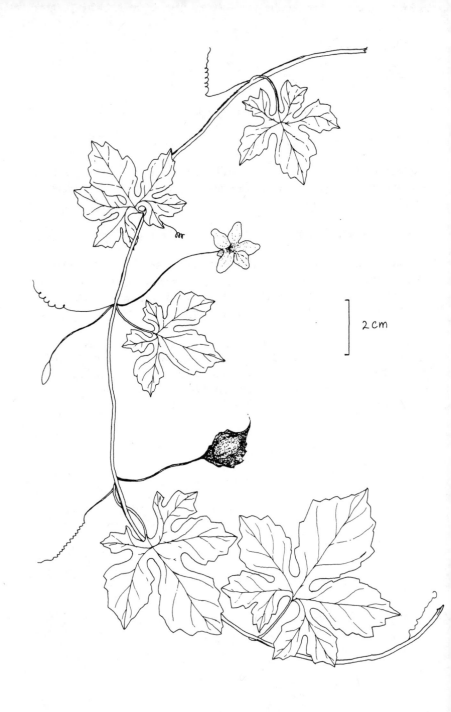

2 cm

Momordica charantia L.

SOROSI (S)

Condiamor (S)

Scientific Name: *Momordica charantia* L.

Plant Family: Cucurbitaceae

Description: Vine growing to 1-2 m tall with a delicate, much-branched stem; leaf deeply lobed; flowers yellow; fruits green, turning yellow-orange when mature; seeds in a red pulp.

Habitat: Clearings, edge of forests, fields, pastures, backyards, empty lots.

Traditional Uses: The most renowned medicinal plant of Belize. Used by grannies and mothers as household tonic to treat and prevent *intestinal parasites, amoebas, anemia, tiredness, constipation, delayed menses, skin problems*, and *painful periods* -- boil small handful of leaves and vine in 3 cups of water for 10 minutes; drink 3 cups daily before meals. Entire plant is boiled to bathe *skin conditions, infections, infestations of ticks and chiggers*, and stubborn *sores* and *wounds* -- boil a large double handful per gallon of water for 15 minutes and allow to cool to tepid. Said to be useful to treat early stages of *diabetes* and is a fine *blood and organ cleanser*. Fresh, raw leaves are chewed for *sore throat* and *mouth sores*.

A related cultivar of this plant is the well known "bitter melon" used in Oriental cuisine. East Indians of Belize relish the ripe fruits in curry dishes.

Research Results: There has been a great deal of pharmacological research on this plant and the resulting literature is quite complex and sometimes contradictory. Caution is advised when ingesting this plant, as more than one source points to its toxicity when taken orally, and pregnant women should avoid it completely. Jelliffe et al. (1954) suggested that the use of this plant may be associated with the development of acute veno-occlusive disease of the liver in Jamaican children. The TRAMIL 4 workshop classified the internal use of the fruit as toxic, but suggested that external use of the leaves and stems was worthy of further investigation (Robineau 1991). Antihyperglycemic activity in humans was demonstrated with an oral dose of the fruit (Leatherdale et al. 1981).

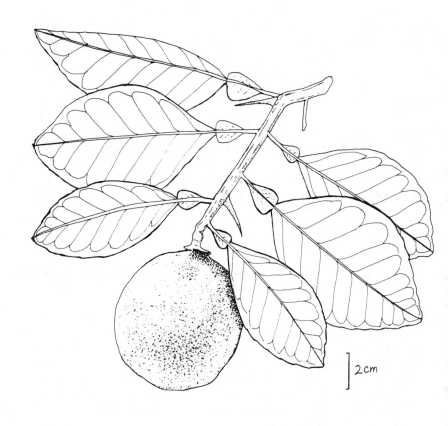

Citrus aurantium L.

2cm

SOUR ORANGE TREE

Naranja Agria (S)
Zutz Pakal (M)

Scientific Name: *Citrus aurantium* L.

Plant Family: Rutaceae

Description: Tree growing to 4 m, with dark brown to black, thorny stems; leaves waxy, green, giving off an aroma of orange oil; flowers white and very aromatic; fruits green, sour to bitter tasting, ca. 7-8 cm in diameter.

Habitat: Yards, edge of forests, roadsides.

Traditional Uses: Semi-cultivated for its wide range of medicinal uses. The leaves, flowers, peel, and juice of the fruit are used in numerous home remedies. Boil 9 leaves in 3 cups of water for 2 minutes; steep 10 minutes and drink 1 cup before each meal for *colds, flu, fever, blood clots, diarrhea, infant colic* or *vomiting* (only 1 cup daily), and *indigestion*. For acute attacks of *indigestion*, simply chew on a leaf, swallowing the juices -- this gives quick relief. Steep a small handful of flowers in 2 cups of boiling water for 20 minutes; strain and drink slowly for *nervousness, hysteria*, and *insomnia*. Steep the rind of 1 fruit in 3 cups of hot water for 20 minutes; strain and drink 1 cup before each meal for *coughs, colds, bronchitis, mucus congestion*, and *indigestion*. Rind may be dried and preserved. Fresh fruit juice is consumed for *liver complaints,* to increase the *appetite*, and as a *general tonic*. For *high blood pressure,* drink 2-3 tablespoons of fresh fruit juice in morning for 10 days.

It is thought that carrying a very young, green fruit in one's pocket will ward off *witchcraft, envy*, and the *evil eye*.

Research Results: This plant has been extensively studied, although many reports in the literature discuss it as a component of herbal mixtures. Thus, it is hard to ascribe the success of the remedy specifically to this plant. The essential oil showed *in vitro* antifungal activity against *Lentinus lepideus, Lenzites trabea,* and *Polyporus versicolor* (Maruzzella et al. 1960). Fresh essential oil (undiluted) showed *in vitro* antibacterial activity against *Pseudomonas aeruginosa* and *Staphylococcus aureus*, and was inactive against *Bacillus cereus* and *Escherichia coli* (Ross et al. 1980). Essential oil from the leaf showed strong *in vitro* antifungal activity against *Aspergillus aegyptiacus, Penicillium cyclopium,* and *Trichoderma viride* (El-Keltawi et al. 1980).

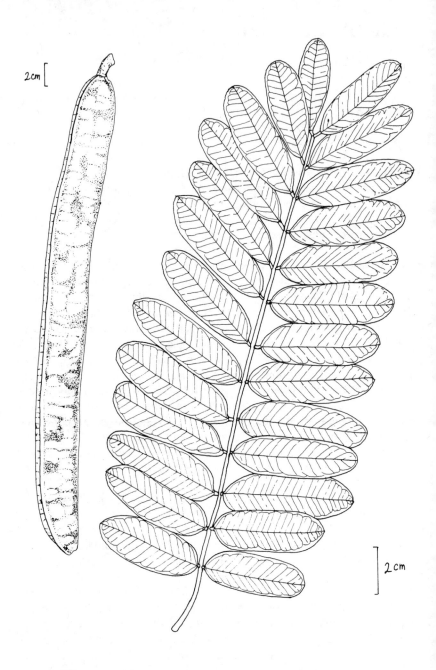

2cm

2 cm

Senna grandis L.

STINKING TOE

Carqué (S)
Bukut (M)

Scientific Name: *Senna grandis* L.

Plant Family: Caesalpiniaceae

Description: Large tree to 30 m tall, with a large, spreading crown; trunk thick, up to 1 m in diameter; leaves with 8-20 pairs of leaflets, each 3-5 cm long; flowers pink or white, in racemes that often appear when the tree has lost most of its leaves; fruits prominent, 30-80 cm long x 2-2.5 cm wide, foul smelling (hence the name "stinking toe").

Habitat: Open fields, pastures, forests.

Traditional Uses: Dark juice of pod is taken as a tonic drink for *anemia, tiredness, malaise* -- remove seeds from pods, strain juice and mix with 50% water or milk; drink 1 cup daily. Juice of fresh leaves is applied to *ringworm, fungus,* or other *skin problems.* For *kidney complaints, water retention, backache,* or *biliousness,* boil 3 small branches with leaves in 3 cups water for 10 minutes and drink in sips all day in place of water. One half cup of fresh leaves infused in 3 cups water and consumed will serve as a *diuretic* and eliminate *toxins* from the body tissue. An infusion of young leaves is used for *diabetes.* For a mild *laxative* and *blood tonic,* boil 1/2 cup fresh leaves in 1 cup water for 2 minutes and drink.

Research Results: A dozen or so chemicals, in various classes including quinoids (Srivastava and Gupta 1981), lignans (López and Hernández 1981), flavonoids (Srivastava and Gupta 1981), carbohydrates (Bose and Srivastava 1978), proteids (Pongpan et al. 1983), and oxygen heterocycle (Kritsanapan 1978) have been found in the leaf, seeds, fruits, and twigs of this species. Little is known of this species' biological activity.

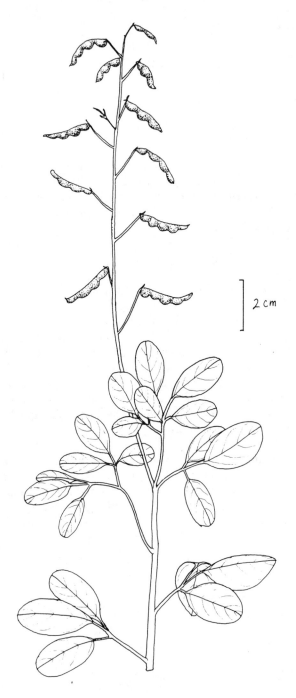

Desmodium adscendens (Sw.) DC.

STRONG BACK

Scientific Name: *Desmodium adscendens* (Swartz) DC.

Plant Family: Fabaceae

Description: Perennial herb, multi-branched, usually prostrate but sometimes erect to 50 cm tall; leaves with 3 leaflets, each 1-3 cm long; inflorescences slender, with numerous light purple flowers; fruit a legume, ca. 3 cm long.

Habitat: Pastures, roadsides, yards.

Traditional Uses: Soak the entire plant in rum for 24 hours and use as a cordial for relief of *backache*; take 1/4 glass 3 times daily for 7-10 days. Boil 1 entire plant in 3 cups water for 10 minutes; drink 1 cup of warm tea before meals for 3-5 days for relief of *backache, muscle pains, kidney ailments*, and *impotency*. Use decoction of entire plant to bathe head to relieve *headaches*; bathe body to relieve *joint aches*.

Research Results: In Ghana and Sierra Leone, the plant is used in traditional medicine to treat asthma (Macfoy and Sama 1983). When the use of this plant against asthma was studied in Ghana, 1-2 teaspoonfuls of dry powder given in 3 divided doses daily prevented asthma in an adult (Ampofo 1977). In guinea pigs, antispasmodic activity was observed from a hot water extract of an unspecified part of this plant (Addy and Dzandu 1986).

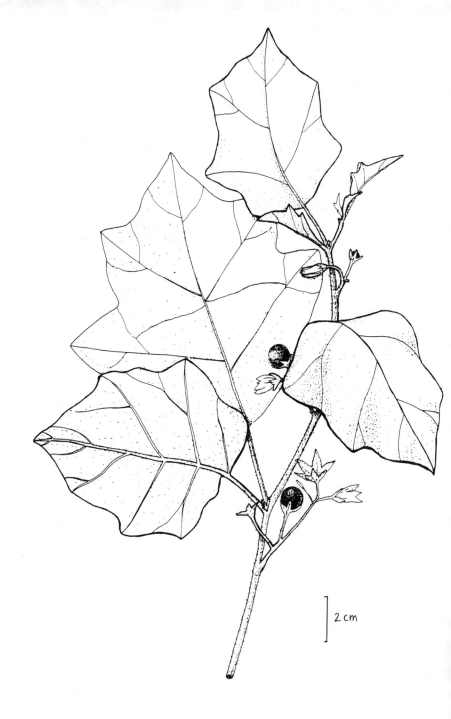

Solanum rudepannum Dunal

SUSUMBA (S)

Pa-al, Toom-pa'ap (M)

Scientific Name: *Solanum rudepannum* Dunal

Plant Family: Solanaceae

Description: Shrub to 4 m with a stem to 3 cm in diameter; leaves deeply lobed, 6-25 cm long, with thorns on underside; flowers small, white, 2-3 cm long; fruit a round, green berry, 1-1.5 cm across.

Habitat: Old fields, pastures, disturbed forests.

Traditional Uses: Used alone, or in combination with other remedies, as a bath for *burns* or *infections of the skin*, and as a tea for *coughs* and *flu*. For both, boil 3 small branches with leaves in 3 cups water for 5 minutes. As tea, drink 1 cup before meals.

For *snakebite*, mashed root is said to be used by snake doctors as a poultice, and boiled leaf as a hot bath. Crush fruits and rub juice on *athlete's foot* to stop itching and eliminate this condition.

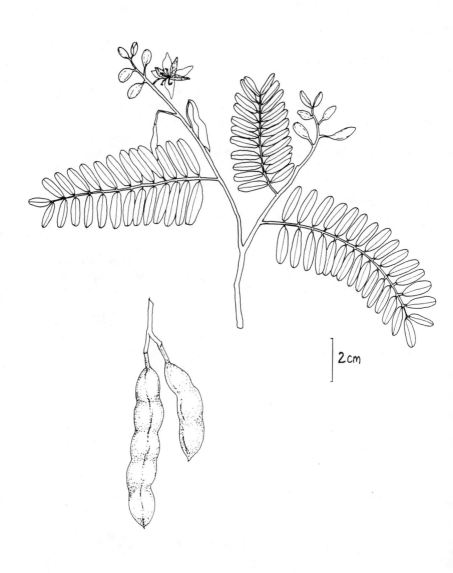

Tamarindus indica L.

TAMARIND

Tamarindo (S)

Scientific Name: *Tamarindus indica* L.

Plant Family: Caesalpiniaceae

Description: Tree to 15-20 m tall, with a stem diameter to 20 cm; fruit a legume, 5-20 cm long, brown, crescent-shaped.

Habitat: Cultivated and naturalized.

Traditional Uses: The pulp of ripe tamarind fruit is soaked in water and used as a *laxative* and to relieve *biliary colic*. It contains calcium, phosphorous, and iron and is, therefore, a fine *cleansing food*. For *morning sickness*, chew a piece of pulp with a dash of salt and pepper. An infusion of the leaves is gargled for *sore throat* and to wash *wounds, boils*, and *rashes*, while a paste of the leaves is applied over *scabies*. Dry and powder leaves to sprinkle over *boils* and *ulcers* of the skin. The bark is astringent and, therefore, is useful as a gargle for *sore throat*. Its powder can be dusted onto *ulcers*; mashed into a paste, it makes a good dressing for *scorpion bite*. Sleeping under a tamarind tree is said to cause ill health.

Research Results: An extract of bark has shown antifugal activity in *Neurospora crassa* (95% ethanol; 50% concentration) (López Abraham et al. 1981). *In vitro* activity against Ranikhet virus was obtained using an ethanol and water (1:1) extract at a concentration of 50 mcg/ml (Dhar et al., 1968). Antibacterial activity using an ethanol (95%) extract of the fruit in agar plate was shown against *Bacillus subtilis, Escherichia coli, Salmonella typhosa, Staphylococcus aureus*, and *Vibrio cholera* (Ray and Majumdar 1976). *In vitro* antischistosomal activity was shown using a water extract of dried fruit at a concentration of 100 PPM in *Schistosoma mansoni* (Elsheikh et al. 1990). Many other positive results for activity as an antiviral, antifungal, and antibacterial were reported in the literature.

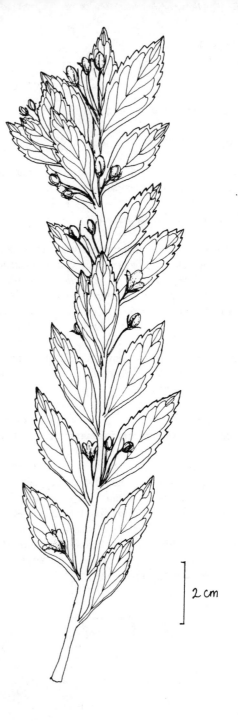

2 cm

Capraria biflora L.

TAN CHI (M)

Pasmo, Pasmo-wa-xi-uil (M)

Scientific Name: *Capraria biflora* L.

Plant Family: Scrophulariaceae

Description: Herb to 1 1/2 m; leaves small, dense, finely toothed; flowers white, ca. 1 cm long, forming in the axils of the leaves.

Habitat: Old fields, pastures; also found on the cayes.

Traditional Uses: For "pasmo," a condition of *blood stagnation* or *congestion* anywhere in the body -- boil two large entire plants in 2 gallons water for 10 minutes and bathe affected area at bedtime; wrap up warmly.

Boil small handful of fresh leaves in 3 cups water for 10 minutes and sip all day to relieve *rheumatic aches and pains*, conditions of the *kidney* or *bladder, cough, tiredness*, and *diabetes*. Also used for *menstrual cramps*, especially in young girls. Considered a tonic herb helpful to all conditions when taken as a tea or a bath.

Research Results: A water extract of dried leaves showed hypoglycemic activity in mice (Pérez et al. 1984). Cytotoxic activity in cell culture against 9KB cancer was seen from a dried root extract (Nascimento et al. 1985). The alkaloid biflorine was isolated from the root (Lima and D'Albuquerque 1958).

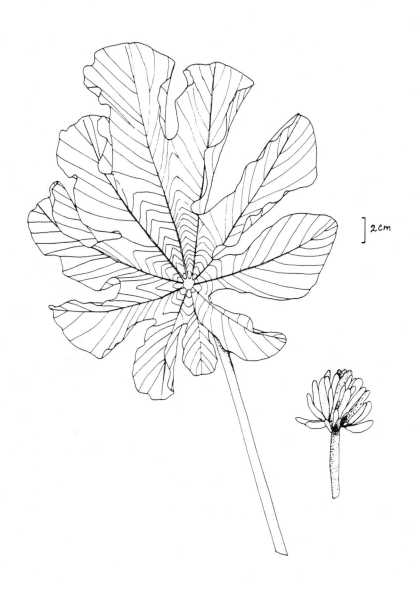

]2cm

Cecropia peltata L.

TRUMPET TREE

Guarumo (S)
Cho-Otz (M)

Scientific Name: *Cecropia peltata* L.

Plant Family: Cecropiaceae

Description: Narrow trunked tree growing to 20 m; bark whitish or gray; leaves lobed; flowers in clusters of 2-6 pinkish-white succulent spikes.

Habitat: Secondary forests, clearings, roadsides, pastures, and other disturbed areas.

Traditional Uses: A leaf infusion is used for *high blood pressure, dropsy,* and *diabetes,* as a *diuretic,* and for a *sedative* effect -- 1 leaf is steeped for 20 minutes in 2 cups hot water; 1 cup of this tea is consumed twice daily for 3 days. A good *liver tonic,* especially when combined with raw papaya in the diet. The tea is useful for *kidney* complaints and *internal infections.* For *sore throat,* use the tea as a gargle. Leaves are boiled 5 minutes and used as a bath to reduce *swellings,* and placed on forehead to reduce *fevers.* A steam bath of leaves is helpful for *rheumatic conditions.*

The dried, powdered leaves make an excellent smoking tobacco used by *chicleros* amd bushmasters.

Research Results: There has been a limited amount of research on the trumpet tree. A dried leaf extract in 95% ethanol has been shown to exhibit *in vitro* antifungal activity against *Neurospora crassa* (López Abraham et al. 1981). A 95% ethanol extract of dried stem exhibited antifungal activity against *Neurospora crassa* at a 50% concentration, while acetone and water extractions were inactive (ibid.). Fresh leaf was shown to be toxic in mice at a minimum dose of 1 ml/animal (95% ethanol extract) and similar results were obtained from a water extract (Feng et al. 1962). In view of the depth of ethnomedical uses and indication of toxicity, further study of this plant seems warranted.

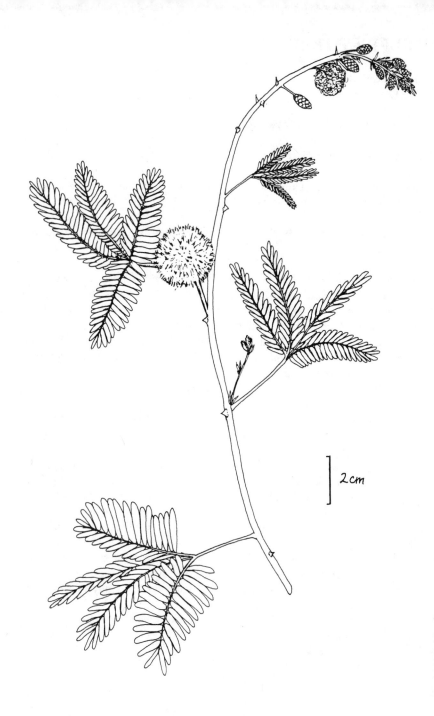

Mimosa pudica L.

TWELVE O'CLOCK

Dormilón (S)
Xmutz (M)

Scientific Name: *Mimosa pudica* L.

Plant Family: Mimosaceae

Description: Low herbaceous plant to 20 cm tall, spreading to 60 cm; stems thorny; leaves pinnate, with 15-25 pairs of pinnae, each 5-10 mm long and folding up when touched; flowers fluffy, mauve.

Habitat: Old fields, roadsides, pastures, and other disturbed sites.

Traditional Uses: As an *antispasmodic, diuretic, relaxant, pain reliever, sleep inducer* -- boil 9 branches with leaves in 3 cups water for 5 minutes; drink 1/2 cup 3-6 times daily as needed. Boil and mash root to apply as poultice to *toothaches*. For *insomnia*, place bunches of leaves under pillow in a cross formation -- 4 crosses for children and 9 for adults. Dry leaves in oven at approximately 100 degrees; remove from stems and powder lightly -- this may be smoked as tobacco to relieve *muscle spasms, backache*, and *nervous irritability*. This same powder may be sprinkled on food as a *sedative*.

Research Results: Antispasmodic activity was obtained in a guinea pig ileum from an ethanol-water (1:1) extract of the entire plant (at an unspecified concentration) (Bhakuni et al. 1969). Antiviral activity was shown in cell culture from an ethanol-water (1:1) extract at a concentration of 50 mcg/ml against *Vaccinia* virus (ibid.). An ethanol-water (1:1) extract of the dried entire plant was active against *Staphylococcus aureus* in an agar plate screen (Avirutnant and Pongpan 1983). Various other antibacterial stems were inactive using this plant. Anti-inflammatory activity was shown in human adults (extract not indicated; dose variable) (Agrawal and Kapadia 1982). The plant is known to contain epinephrine adrenalin (Applewhite 1973).

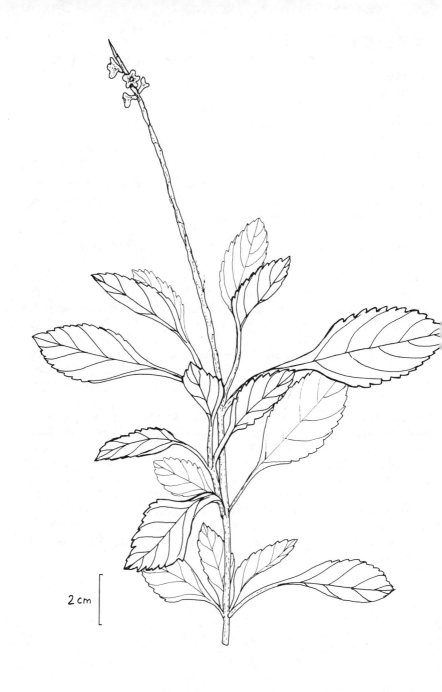

Stachytarpheta cayennensis (L. Rich.) Vahl.

VERVAIN

Vervine (E)
Verbena (S)
Cot-acam (M)

Scientific Name: *Stachytarpheta cayennensis* (L. Rich.) Vahl.

Plant Family: Verbenaceae

Description: Herbaceous plant growing to about 1 m tall; leaves opposite with toothed margins, 3-10 cm long; flowers purple, 7-10 mm long, borne on long spikes 10-40 cm long, appearing throughout most of the year.

Habitat: Old fields, edge of forest, backyards, roadsides.

Traditional Uses: Considered sacred by the Maya and still used in ritual ceremonies to ward off evil influences. Bunches of stems are hung in doorways to repel *witchcraft* and dried leaves are burned as incense.

Tea is drunk for *nervousness, heart conditions, stomachache, neuralgia, cough, colds, fever, flu*, and *liver* complaints -- boil 3 branches about 15 cm long with leaves in 3 cups water for 5 minutes; drink 1 cup before each meal. This is a very cooling herb that is useful in *feverish states* and for *overexposure to sun or heat*. Mashed leaves are applied as a healing poultice to *boils* and *infected sores*. For *intestinal parasites* of adults, take 1/4 cup of fresh leaf juice daily for 7 days and re-test stool.

Midwives use entire plant to make a steam bath for vaginal parts after *childbirth* to prevent *infection* and to insure that *womb* returns to proper position. Also, a tea of leaves is administered as a douche for *gonorrhea* and to postpartum women to *cleanse uterus*.

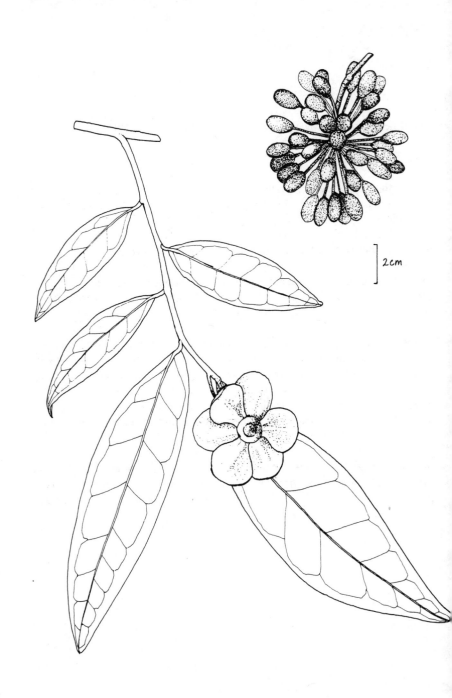

2cm

Malmea depressa (Baillon) R.E. Fries

WILD COFFEE

Eremuil (S)

Scientific Name: *Malmea depressa* (Baillon) R. E. Fries

Plant Family: Annonaceae

Description: Small tree to 5 m tall; leaves dark green, aromatic; flowers greenish; fruits in small clusters, turning red-orange when ripe.

Habitat: Primary and disturbed forests.

Traditional Uses: This is a very effective plant for bathing those with *fever, insomnia, malaise, backache, arthritis, rheumatism, nervousness*, or *skin ailments* -- boil a quart-sized container of fresh leaves in 2 gallons of water for 10 minutes; allow the mixture to become warm, not hot, and bathe patient.

Wild coffee can also be used as a tea to treat *hysteria, nervousness, insomnia, menstrual cramps*, and *headaches* -- boil 9 fresh leaves in 3 cups of water for 5 minutes and serve.

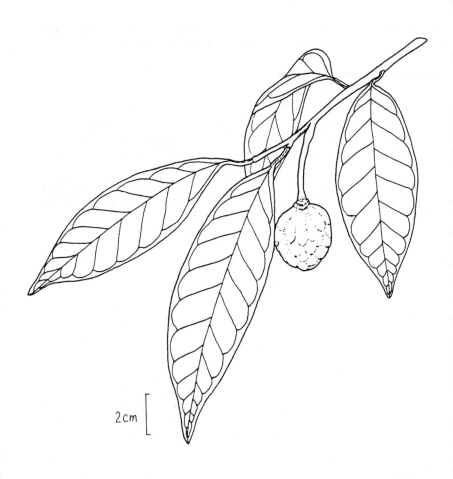

2cm

Annona reticulata L.

WILD CUSTARD APPLE

Anona (S)

Scientific Name: *Annona reticulata* L.

Plant Family: Annonaceae

Description: Tree to 10 m in height or more; leaves to 20 cm long; fruit heart-shaped, green in color, turning reddish-yellow or brown when ripe, 10 cm in diameter, and smooth to the touch.

Habitat: Forests, fields, riversides.

Traditional Uses: An excellent food and medicinal tree, used since pre-conquest times. All parts of the tree are useful.

The ripe fruit is small and seedy with a pleasant aroma and flavor. Raw fruit pulp can be used as a dressing for *boils* to hasten pus formation. Apply pounded seeds as a poultice to scalp to treat *head lice* and *dandruff* -- wrap head in scarf and leave on overnight.

The leaves are cooling and are tied to soles of the feet to lower *fever*. Wash *mouth sores* with leaf tea. Apply leaf to temples and forehead to reduce *headaches* and *fevers*. Rub fresh leaf juice on *plantars' warts* for 9 days. Cook leaf a few minutes in oil and apply to *swellings* and *bruises*. Soak leaf in alcohol and use this mixture to massage *feverish persons* to lower temperature by drawing out heat. Mashed bark with a pinch of salt is an excellent healing poultice for *sprains*, *strains*, and *fractures*; wrap the injury securely in cloth and change poultice daily. Boil fresh leaves with sugar to make a *cough* syrup. A bath for *skin conditions* is made by boiling the fresh leaves in water.

Research Results: This plant has been tested extensively in the area of pheromones, insecticidal activity, and feeding deterrant activity, with a great deal of success. For example, Atal et al. (1978) report that the dried aerial parts of this plant in an ethanol-water mixture at 1% concentration showed insecticidal activity against *Tribolium castaneum* (flour beetle). Feeding deterrant activity against lesser rice weevils was shown in an acetone extract of dried seeds (Islam 1984). This plant family is rich in chemicals and this species, in particular, has been found to contain indole alkaloids (Yang and Cheng 1987), isoquinoline alkaloids, lactones (Saad et al. 1991), sesquiterpenes, diterpenes (Oguntimein 1987), and leucoanthocyanins (Narayana et al. 1981).

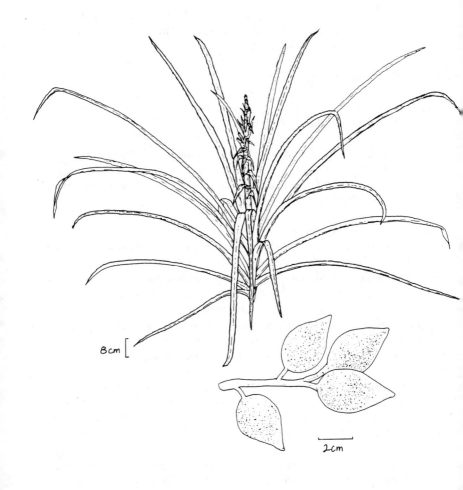

8cm

2cm

Bromelia pinguin L.

WILD PINEAPPLE

Piñuelo (S)
Ix-Tot (M)

Scientific Name: *Bromelia pinguin* L.

Plant Family: Bromeliaceae

Description: Pineapple-like plant; leaves long, hooked, thorny, to 2 m long, sometimes tinged with red at center and tips; inflorescences on long spikes arising from center of plant; flowers to 6 cm long, rose-white-green in color; fruit a tubular berry, yellow, acidic, aromatic, and edible.

Habitat: Forests.

Traditional Uses: Pound leaves with salt to use as a poultice for *sprains, fractures*, or *broken bones* -- apply directly to afflicted area.

Research Results: An aqueous extract of the fresh leaf was shown to have hypotensive activity in dogs and smooth muscle relaxant activity in rabbits (Feng et al. 1962). The same study reported similar results in rabbits from an ethanol extract, as well as spasmolytic activity in guinea pigs. Finally, this study reported vasodilator activity in rats using an ethanol extract of leaves. A methanol extract of dried root and stem of wild pineapple showed *in vitro* cytotoxic activity (Raffauf et al. 1981). This species has been found to contain lipids, flavonoids, lignans, and diterpenes in the root and stem (ibid. 1981).

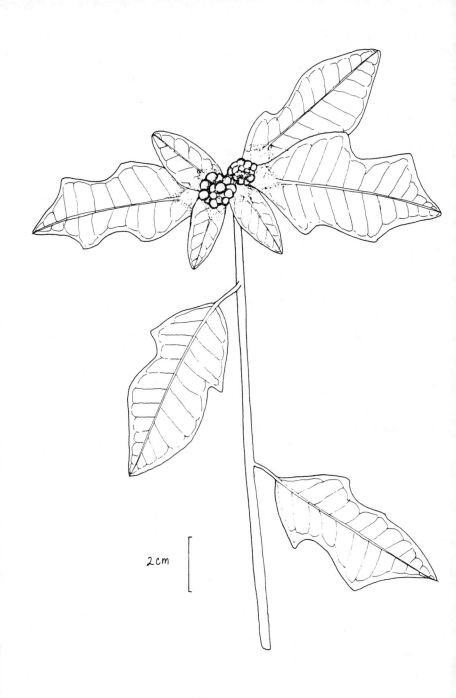

2cm

Euphorbia pulcherrima Willd. ex Klotzsch

WILD POINSETTIA

Flor de Pascua del Monte (S)

Scientific Name: *Euphorbia pulcherrima* Willd. ex Klotzsch

Plant Family: Euphorbiaceae

Description: Shrub to 1-4 m tall, with upright green stems; leaves 12-20 cm long, green; inflorescence of large, reddish bracts surrounding small, green-yellow flowers.

Habitat: Weed in old fields.

Traditional Uses: To *increase the flow of mother's milk* and to relieve *swollen breasts*, braid 9 of these plants in a necklace and have the mother wear this for 3 days. Also, boil 9 entire plants in a gallon of water for 10 minutes and bathe breasts in this warm tea twice daily. According to Standley and Steyermark (1949), poultices made from the leaves are applied to relieve *body pains* and the milk of the stem is used as a *depilatory*. The plant is quite toxic if taken internally.

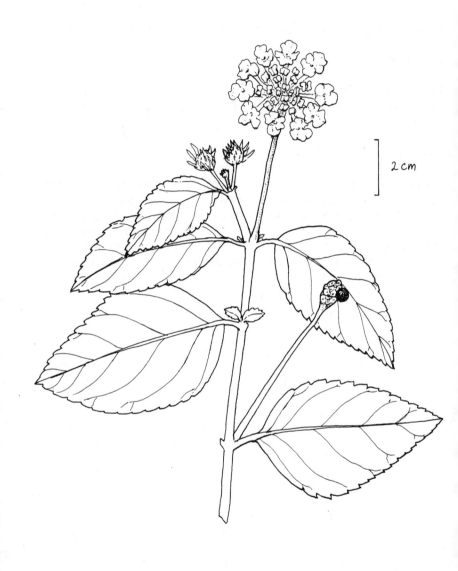

2 cm

Lantana camara L.

WILD SAGE

Scientific Name: *Lantana camara* **L.**

Plant Family: Verbenaceae

Description: Shrub to 1-3 m in height, spreading; leaves 2-12 cm long, with serrated margins and a strong odor when crushed; flowers in dense heads, yellow to orange, changing to red or purple, each flower 2-6 mm across; fruit a drupe, turning blue to black when ripe, shiny, and full of juice.

Habitat: Cultivated shrub common in gardens, old fields, roadsides, trails.

Traditional Uses: The leaves are used to relieve *itching*, either by making a powder from dried leaves and applying it directly to the affected area or by bathing in a leaf infusion. While there are numerous traditional uses that involve ingestion of the leaf, the TRAMIL 4 workshop states that this plant is toxic and should not be taken internally (Robineau 1991).

Research Results: This is a widely used and well-studied plant. It is a troublesome weed from the standpoint of livestock farmers, inducing photosensitivity in sheep, cattle and other animals and proving toxic when ingested (Kingsbury 1964). The primary substance responsible is a polycyclic triterpenoid named lantadene A (Louw 1948). Children eating the berries have been poisoned, exhibiting muscular weakness, circulatory collapse and, in lesser cases, gastrointestinal irritation (Verhulst and Page 1962). In an *in vitro* study, the essential oil has shown antibacterial activity against *Pseudomonas aeruginosa* and *Staphylococcus aureus* (Ross et al. 1980). An extract of dried leaves has shown antifungal activity against *Aspergillus fumigatus* and *Aspergillus niger* (Saksena and Tripathi 1985). In humans, a leaf paste exhibited antihemorrhagic activity, effective on wounds in 80% of cases studied (Wanjari 1983). As the pharmacological literature is abundant with cases of toxicity in animals (e.g., hepatotoxic activity, nephrotoxic activity, etc.), caution is advised when using this plant.

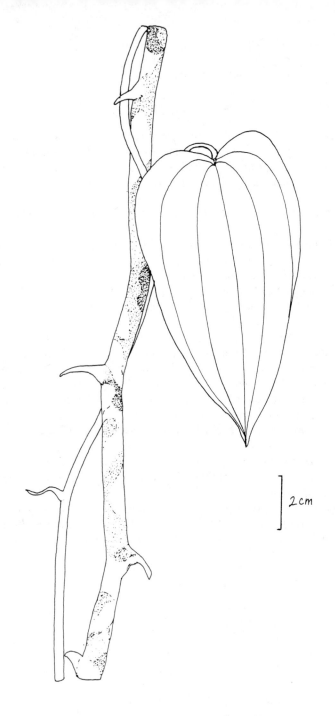

]2 cm

Dioscorea aff. *belizensis* Lundell

WILD YAM

Cocolmeca, Barba del Viejo (S)

Scientific Name: *Dioscorea* aff. *belizensis* Lundell

Plant Family: Dioscoreaceae

Description: Small to large vine with knotty, tuberous root; stems several, thick, green, thorny; leaves heart-shaped, emerging and turning green when mature; flowers dark red; fruits dark brown.

Habitat: Moist forests.

Traditional Uses: Popular household remedy for ailments of the urinary tract such as *bladder infections, stoppage of urine,* and *kidney sluggishness* and *malfunction* -- boil a small handful of chopped root in 3 cups of water for 10 minutes; consume 3 cups taken in sips throughout the day. To *loosen mucus* in *coughs* and *colds*, to reduce *fevers*, to relieve *bilious colic*, to *build the blood*, to relieve the pains of *rheumatism* and *arthritis*, and for the onset of *diabetes*, prepare a hot tea made from the tuber and drink 3 times daily before meals. To prevent *miscarriages*, mix chopped root with fresh grated ginger and take as tea 3 times daily. For *impotency* in men, soak wild yam in gin for 10 days and take 1 tablespoon 3 times daily. For *infertility* in women, soak wild yam in "anisado" (anise liqueur) for 10 days and take 3 tablespoons daily.

Research Results: The tuber of *Dioscorea belizensis* is known to contain steroids and triterpenes. A closely related species, *Dioscorea mexicana* (Mexican Yam), contains diosgenin, a steroid precursor which can be converted to progesterone and then synthesized. This discovery enabled the development of synthetic hormones, useful, for example, in the birth control pill (Griggs 1981).

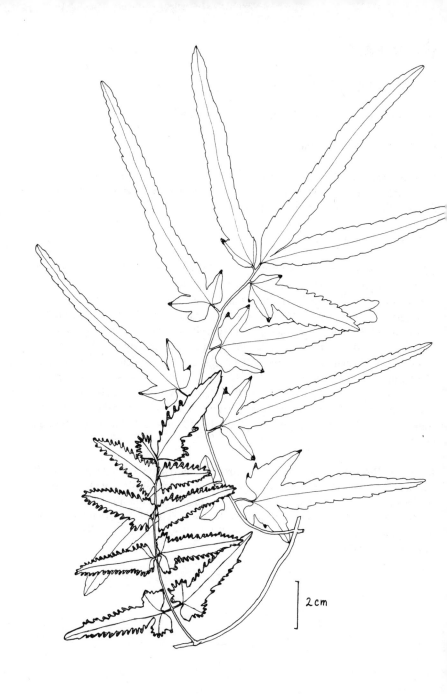

Lygodium venustum Sw.

WIRE WIS

Behuco de Alhambre (S)
Alambre Xiv (S, M)
Xix-el-ba (M)

Scientific Name: *Lygodium venustum* Sw.

Plant Family: Schizaeaceae

Description: A vining fern that creeps along the ground and also climbs onto other plants, growing to ca. 2.5 m high; leaves serrated, pinnate to bipinnate, to 25 cm long and 20 cm wide, smaller towards apex, with brown sori (spore capsules) on edges of leaves.

Habitat: Old fields, clearings, pastures, disturbed forest.

Traditional Uses: To treat *skin fungus*, boil a large double handful of leaves in 1 quart of water for 10 minutes; soak affected area in very hot mixture twice daily. Apply fresh plant juice to *sores, rashes*, and *skin conditions*. A poultice can be made from the leaves and applied to head for *headache*.

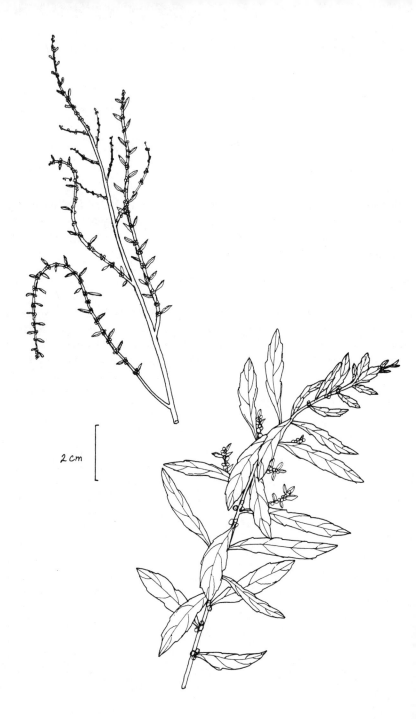

Chenopodium ambrosioides L.

WORMSEED

Mexican Weed (E)
Epazote (S)

Scientific Name: *Chenopodium ambrosioides* L.

Plant Family: Chenopodiaceae

Description: Herb to 1 m, many branched; leaves small, ovate or lanceolate, sharply toothed; flowers green, formed in dense spikes. Leaves and stems are highly aromatic.

Habitat: A weedy species found near houses, in fields, and in other disturbed sites.

Traditional Uses: A popular household remedy used to rid children and adults of *intestinal parasites* -- 1 teaspoon of the juice of mashed leaves is given in 1/2 cup warm milk or taken alone for 3 consecutive mornings prior to eating; on the fourth day, give 1 tablespoon castor oil; have the person use a chamber pot and observe what passes in the stool. Hot leaf tea is taken as a *sedative* -- boil 3 small branches in 1 cup water. The root of 1 large plant boiled in 2 cups of water for 10 minutes and drunk hot is an excellent remedy for "crudo" or *hangover*. Epazote is added to beans for a delightful flavor and, eaten raw, eliminates *intestinal gas* and aids *digestion*. This plant should not be given to pregnant women, the weak, or the aged.

Research Results: A great deal of research has been carried out on this widely used plant. It has been associated with many poisonings, usually due to overdoses of the oil, which have proven fatal to humans (Kingsbury 1964). According to this author, fatalities from "the natural ingestion of the plant do not appear to have occured except possibly in geese." (p. 234). Photosensitization has also been noted in a woman working in a field of this plant. Symptoms included edema of face, hands, and feet, and extravasations with skin necrosis. Treatments with ACTH, cortisone, vitamin C, and antihistamines were effective (Lubieniecki 1961). The essential oil has shown *in vitro* antifungal activity against *Absidia ramosa, Microsporum gypsum*, and *Trichophyton mentagrophytes* at a concentration of 1000 PPM (Kishore et al. 1981). A water extract of the plant, when given to rats in a dose of 10 mg/kg showed carcinogenic activity, with 11 of 15 rats developing tumors (Ahmad et al. 1979). Antiascariasis (*Ascaris lumbricoides*) was demonstrated *in vitro* with a 0.5 gm/liter concentration of essential oil (Ali and Mehta 1970).

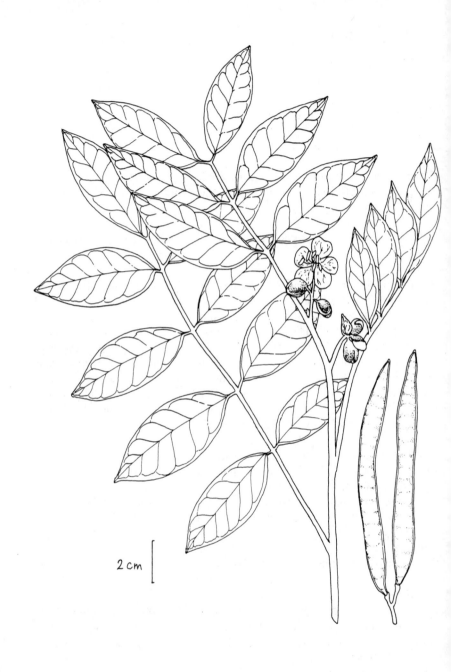

2 cm

Senna occidentalis (L.) Link

YAMA BUSH

Rat Bean (E)
Frijolillo (S)

Scientific Name: *Senna occidentalis* (L.) Link

Plant Family: Caesalpiniaceae

Description: A weedy annual herb to 1 m tall with stout branches; leaves with 4-6 pairs of leaflets, each 3-7 cm long; flowers in yellow racemes arising from the leaf axils; fruit a pod, 6-12 cm long x 6-9 mm wide.

Habitat: Clearings, edge of forests, roadside, pastures, yards, empty lots.

Traditional Uses: Useful as a tonic herb for many ailments -- make tea from entire plant boiled for 10 minutes in 3 cups water and drink 2 cups daily. One root is boiled with 2 cups of water for 10 minutes and consumed warm twice daily for *fever* and *flu*. Leaves are toasted, ground, and mixed with egg white and brandy to be applied as a poultice to pulse at wrist of child or adult to counteract *weakness* and *exhaustion* (especially due to old age or illness). Midwives do a *pregnancy test* by having women urinate on yama bush leaves; if leaves look scorched, baby is due. For *menstrual pain,* boil roots of 1 plant in 3 cups of water for 10 minutes; drink 3 cups hot before meals. For *weakness of heart*, mash leaves with egg and rum; wrap this in cotton cloth and lay over heart against skin once daily for 1 hour. To rid a rude, crabby child of its bad temper, spank the child with branches of this plant; then throw the branches away. The roasted, ground seeds make a fine coffee substitute.

Research Results: There has been a great deal of chemical and pharmacological work with this plant. *In vitro* antifungal activity against *Epidermophyton floccosum, Microsporum gypseum, Trichophyton mentagrophytes,* and *Trichophyton rubrum* has been shown in broth culture from a 1 ml concentration hot water extract of dried root, leaf, and seed (Cáceres et al. 1991). Undiluted essential leaf oil has shown *in vitro* activity against *Fusarium oxysporum* (Pandey et al. 1982). Cardiotoxic activity of seeds was shown in rabbits (O'Hara and Pierce 1974), and toxicity was demonstrated in dogs with an oral dose of dried seed (Moussu 1925). Various other toxic activities have been shown from the seeds. Caution is, therefore, suggested when using this plant and further biomedical evaluation of its potential hazards would seem to be indicated.

REFERENCES

Achenbach, H., H. Grob, and J. Portecop. 1984. Ishwarol, the main sesquiterpene in *Piper amalago*. Planta Med. **50**(6):528-529.

Addy, M.E. and W.K. Dzandu. 1986. Dose-response effects of *Desmodium adscendens* aqueous extract on histamine response, content and anaphylactic reactions in the guinea pig. J. Ethnopharmacol. **18**:13-20.

Agrawal, R.C. and L.A. Kapadia. 1982. Treatment of piles with indigenous drugs: Pilex tablets and ointment along with styplon. Probe **21**(3):201-204.

Ahmad, M.U., S.K. Husain, A.A. Ansari, and S.M. Osman. 1979. Studies on herbaceous seed oils. 12. J. Oil Technol. Assoc. India **11**(3):70-72.

Ajao, A.O., O. Shonukan, and B. Femi-Onadeko. 1985. Antibacterial effect of aqueous and alcohol extracts of *Spondias mombin*, and *Alchornea cordifolia*: Two local antimicrobial remedies. Int. J. Crude Drug Res. **23**(2):67-72.

Akhtar, M.S., Q.M. Khan, and T. Khaliq. 1985. Effects of *Portulaca oleracae [sic]* (Kulfa) and *Taraxacum officinale* (Dhudhal) in normoglycaemic and alloxan-treated hyperglycaemic rabbits. J. Pak. Med. Ass. **35**:207-210.

Ali, S.M. and R.K. Mehta. 1970. Preliminary pharmacological and anthelmintic studies of the essential oil of *Piper betle*. Indian J. Pharmacy. **32**:132-133.

Ampofo, O. 1977. Plants that heal. World Health **1977**:26-30.

Applewhite, P.B. 1973. Serotonin and norepinephrine in plant tissues. Phytochemistry **12**:191.

Atal, C.K., J.B. Srivastava, B.K. Wali, R.B. Chakravarty, B.N. Dhawan, and R.P. Rastogi. 1978. Screening of Indian plants for biological activity. Part VIII. Indian J. Exp. Biol. **16**:330-349.

Athanassova-Shopova, S. and K. Roussinov. 1965. Pharmacological studies of Bulgarian plants with a view to their anti-convulsive effect. Cr. Acad. Bulg. Sci. **18**:691.

Avirutnant, W. and A. Pongpan. 1983. The antimicrobial activity of some Thai flowers and plants. Mahidol Univ. J. Pharm. Sci. **10**(3):81-86.

Awuah, R.T. 1989. Fungitoxic effects of extracts from some West African plants. Ann. Appl. Biol. **115**(3):451-453.

Ayensu, E.S. 1978. *Medicinal plants of the West Indies*. Unpublished manuscript. Washington, DC: Office of Biological Conservat. 110 pp.

_____. 1982. *Medicinal plants of the West Indies*. U.S.A.: Reference Publications. 283 pp.

Aynehchi, Y., M.H. Salehi Sormaghi, G.H. Amin, M. Khoshkhow, and A. Shabani. 1985. Survey of Iranian plants for saponins, alkaloids, flavonoids and tannins. 3. Int. J. Crude Drug Res. **23**(1):33-41.

_____, _____, M. Shirudi, and E. Souri. 1982. Screening of Iranian plants for antimicrobial activity. Acta Pharm. Suecica **19**(4):303-308.

REFERENCES

Bailey, L.H. and E.Z. Bailey. 1976. *Hortus Third: A Concise Dictionary of Plants Cultivated in the United States and Canada.* Revised and expanded by the staff of the Liberty Hyde Bailey Hortorium, New York State College of Agriculture and Life Sciences, State University at Cornell University. New York: Macmillan Publishing Company; London: Collier Macmillan Publishers. 1290 pp.

Barnes, T.C. 1947. The healing action of extracts of *Aloe vera* leaf on abrasions of human skin. Amer. J. Bot. **34**:597.

Barros, G.S.G., F.J.A. Matos, J.E.V. Vieira, M.P. Sousa, and M.C. Medeiros. 1970. Pharmacological screening of some Brazilian plants. J. Pharm. Pharmacol. **22**:116.

Barua, R.N., R.P. Sharma, G. Thyagarajan, and W. Herz. 1978. Flavonoids of *Chromolaena odorata.* Phytochemistry **17**:1807-1808.

Benjamin, T.V. 1980. Analysis of the volatile constituents of local plants used for skin disease. J. Afr. Med. Pl. **1980**:135-139.

Best, R., D.A. Lewis, and N. Nasser. 1984. The anti-ulcerogenic activity of the unripe plantain banana (*Musa* species). Brit. J. Pharmacol. **82**(1):107-116.

Bhakuni, O.S., M.L. Dhar, M.M. Dhar, B.N. Dhawan, and B.N. Mehrotra. 1969. Screening of Indian plants for biological activity. Part 2. Indian J. Exp. Biol. **7**:250-262.

Bohlmann, F., J. Ziesche, R.M. King, and H. Robinson. 1981. Naturally occurring terpene derivatives. Part 300. Eudesmanolides and diterpenes from *Wedelia trilobata* and an ent-kaurenic acid derivative from *Aspilia parvifolia.* Phytochemistry **20**(4):751-756.

_____ and Ngo-Le-Van. 1977. Naturally occurring terpene derivatives. 97. New kaurene derivatives from *Wedelia* species. Phytochemistry **16**(5):579-581.

Bose, S. and H.C. Srivastava. 1978. Structure of a polysaccharide from the seeds of *Cassia grandis* L. Part 1. Hydrolytic studies. Indian J. Chem. Ser. B. **16**:966-969.

Butler, C.L. and L.E. Mullen. 1955. Investigation of *Piscidia erythrina* (Jamaica dogwood). Acta Phytotherap. **2**(8):1.

Cáceres, A., B.R. López, M.A. Girón, and H. Logemann. 1991. Plants used in Guatemala for the treatment of dermatophytic infections. 1. Screening for antimycotic activity of 44 plant extracts. J. Ethnopharmacol. **31**(3):263-276.

_____, L.M. Girón, S.R. Alvarado, and M.F. Torres. 1987. Screening of antimicrobial activity of plants popularly used in Guatemala for the treatment of dermatomucosal diseases. J. Ethnopharmacol. **20**(3):223-237.

Caldwell, M.E. and W.R. Brewer. 1983. Plants with potential to enhance significant tumor growth. Cancer Res. **43**(12):5775-5777.

REFERENCES

Carlini, E.A., J.D.D.P. Contar, A.R. Silva Filho, N.G. Solveira Filho, M.L. Frochtengarten, and O.F.A. Bueno. 1986. Pharmacology of lemongrass (*Cymbopogon citratus* Stapf.). 1. Effects of teas prepared from the leaves on laboratory animals. J. Ethnopharmacol. **17(1)**:37-64.

Chapuis, J.C., B. Sordat, and K. Hostettmann. 1988. Screening for cytotoxic activity of plants used in traditional medicine. J. Ethnopharmacol. **23(2/3)**:273-284.

Cobble, H.H. 1975. Stabilized *Aloe vera* gel. Patent-U.S.-3, 892, 853.

Compadre, C.M. and A.D. Kinghorn. 1985. Studies on the sweet principle of *Lippia dulcis* and on steviol, the aglycone of stevioside. Ph.D. dissertation, University of Illinois at Chicago. 212 pp.

_____, E.F. Robbins, and A.D. Kinghorn. 1986. The intensely sweet herb, *Lippia dulcis* Trev.: Historical uses, field inquiries, and constituents. J. Ethnopharmacol. **15(1)**:89-106.

Corthout, J., J. Totte, M. Claeys, L. Pieters, D. Van Den Berghe, and A.J. Vlietinck. 1985. Antivirally active substances from *Spondias mombin* L. (Anacardiaceae). Abstr. Internat. Res. Cong. Nat. Prod., Coll. Pharm., Univ. N. Carolina, Chapel Hill, N. Carolina, July 7-12, 1985. **Abstr-53.**

Coutts, B.C. 1979. Stabilized *Aloe vera* gel. Patent-Japan Kokai Tokkyo Koho-79 119, 018. 6 pp.

Crewe, J.E. 1939. Aloes in the treatment of burns and scalds. Minnesota Med. **22**:538-539.

Czeczuga, B. 1985. Carotenoids in sixty-six representatives of the Pteridophyta. Biochem. Syst. Ecol. **13(3)**:221-230.

Davis, R.H., W.L. Parker, and D.P. Murdoch. 1991. *Aloe vera* as a biologically active vehicle for hydrocortisone acetate. J. Amer. Pod. Med. Assn. **81(1)**:1-9.

Dayal, R. 1985. Phytochemical investigation on flowers of *Gliricidia sepium*. J. Indian Chem. Soc. **62(2)**:171.

Der Marderosian, A.H., F.B. Giller, and F.C. Roia. 1976. Phytochemical and toxicological screening of household ornamental plants potentially toxic to humans. I. J. Toxicol. Environ. Health. **1**:939.

Dhar, M.L., M.M. Dhar, B.N. Dhawan, B.N. Mehrotra, and C. Ray. 1968. Screening of Indian plants for biological activity. Part 1. Indian J. Exp. Biol. **6**:232-247.

Dhawan, B.N., G.K. Patnaik, R.P. Rastogi, K.K. Singh, and J.S. Tandon. 1977. Screening of Indian plants for biological activity. 6. Indian J. Exp. Biol. **15**:208.

Domínguez S., X.A. and J.B. Alcorn. 1985. Screening of medicinal plants used by Huastec Mayans of Northeastern Mexico. J. Ethnopharmacol. **13(2)**:139-156.

REFERENCES

_____, J. Verde, S. Sucar, and R. Trevino. 1986. Two amides from *Piper amalago*. Phytochemistry **25**(1):239-240.

_____, P. Rojas, M. del R. Garza, and J.A. Córdova. 1962. Preliminary study of 25 plants from the central territory of Quintana Roo, Mexico. Rev. Soc. Quim Mex. **6**:213-215.

Dunham, N.W. and K.R. Allard. 1960. A preliminary pharmacologic investigation of the roots of *Bixa orellana*. J. Amer. Pharm. Ass. Sci. Ed. **49**:218.

Durand, E., E.V. Ellington, P.C. Feng, L.J. Haynes, K.E. Magnus, and N. Philip. 1962. Simple hypotensive and hypertensive principles from some West Indian medicinal plants. J. Pharm. Pharmacol. **14**:562-566.

El-Hafiz, M.A.A., B. Weniger, J.C. Quirion, and R. Anton. 1991. Keto-alcohols, lignans and coumarins from *Chiococca alba*. Phytochemistry **30**(6):2029-2031.

El-Keltawi, N.E.M., S.E. Megalla, and S.A. Ross. 1980. Antimicrobial activity of some Egyptian aromatic plants. Herba Pol. **26**(4):245-250.

Elsheikh, S.H., A.K. Bashir, S.M. Suliman, and M.E. Wassila. 1990. Toxicity of certain Sudanese plant extracts on *Cercariae* and *Miracidia* of *Schistosoma mansoni*. Int. J. Crude Drug Res. **28**(4): 241-245.

Emeruwa, A.C. 1982. Antibacterial substance from *Carica papaya* fruit extract. J. Nat. Prod. **45**:123-127.

Esposito-Avella, M., P. Brown, I. Tejeira, R. Buitrago, L. Barrios, C. Sánchez, M.P. Gupta, and J. Cedeño. 1985. Pharmacological screening of Panamanian medicinal plants. Part 1. Int. J. Crude Drug. Res. **23**(1):17-25.

Farnsworth, N.R. 1993. Personal communication.

Feng, P.C., L.J. Haynes, K.E. Magnus, J.R. Plimmer, and H.S.A. Sherrat. 1962. Pharmacological screening of some West Indian medicinal plants. J. Pharm. Pharmacol. **14**:556-561.

Fernandez, B. 1990. *Medicine Woman: The Herbal Tradition of Belize*. Belize City, Belize: National Library Service. 58 pp.

Fernando, T. and G. Bean. 1985. A comparison of the fatty acids and sterols of seeds of weedy and vegetable species of *Amaranthus* spp. J. Amer. Oil Chem. Soc. **62**(1):89-91.

Fitzpatrick, F.K. 1954. Plant substances active against *Mycobacterium tuberculosis*. Antibiot. Chemother. **4**:528.

Flath, R.A., R.R. Forrey, J.O. John, and B.G. Chan. 1978. Volatile components of corn silk: Possible *Heliothis zea* attractants. J. Agr. Food Chem. **26**:1290.

Freise, F.W. 1935. The occurrence of caffeine in Brazilian medicinal plants. Pharm. Zentralhalle Dtschl. **76**:704-706.

REFERENCES

Frischknecht, P.M., J. Ulmer-Dufek, and T.W. Baumann. 1986. Purine alkaloid formation in buds and developing leaflets of *Coffea arabica*: Expression of an optimal defense strategy? Phytochemistry **25**(3):613-616.

Fuzellier, M.C., F. Mortier, and P. Lectard. 1982. Antifongic *[sic]* activity of *Cassia alata* L.. Ann. Pharm. **40**:357-363.

Galal, E.E., A. Kandil, R. Hegazy, M. El-Ghoroury, and W. Gobran. 1975. *Aloe vera* and gastrogenic ulceration. J. Drug Res. **7**(2):73.

Ganguly, S.N. and S.M. Sircar. 1974. Gibberellins from Mangrove plants. Phytochemistry **13**(9):1911-1913.

George, M. and K.M. Pandalai. 1949. Investigations on plant antibiotics. Part 4. Further search for antibiotic substances in Indian medicinal plants. Indian J. Med. Res. **37**:169-181.

German, V.F.. 1971. Isolation and characterization of cytotoxic principles from *Hyptis verticillata*. J. Pharm. Sci. **60**:649.

Gilfillan, W.. 1862. The leaves of the *Ricinus communis*, as a galactagogue. Amer. Med. Times. **4**:218.

Gómez, L.D. and J.W. Wallace. 1986. Flavonoids of *Phlebodium*. Biochem. Syst. Ecol. **14**(4):407-408.

González, F. and M. Silva. 1987. A survey of plants with antifertility properties described in the South American folk medicine. Abstr. Princess Congress I, Bangkok Thailand, 10-13 December, 1987. 20 pp.

González, J., R. Noriega, and R. Sandoval. 1975. Contribution to the study of flavonoids of coffee tree (*Coffea*) leaves. Re. Colomb. Quim. **5**:289.

Goyal, M.M. and K. Kumar. 1987. Alkyl sterols in the leaves of *Lagerstroemia indica*. Bangladesh J. Sci. Ind. Res. **22**(1/4):148-151.

Griffiths, L.A. 1959. On the distribution of gentisic acid in green plants. J. Exp. Biol. **10**:437.

Griggs, B. 1981. *Green Pharmacy*. London: Jill Norman & Hobhouse Ltd.

Gupta, M.P., N.G. Solis, M. Esposito-Avella, and C. Sánchez. 1984. Hypoglycemic activity of *Neurolaena lobata* (L.) R.Br.. J. Ethnopharmacol. **10**(3):323-327.

Harborne, J.B. 1975. Flavonoid bisulphates and their co-occurences with ellagic acid in the Bixaceae, Frankeniaceae and related families. Phytochemistry **14**:1331.

Heal, R.E., E.F. Rogers, R.T. Wallace, and O. Starnes. 1950. A survey of plants for insecticidal activity. Lloydia **13**:89-162.

Hegnauer, R. 1963. *Chemotaxonomy der Pflanzen*. Bäle et Stuttgart: Birkhauser Verlag. 540 pp.

Heskel, N.S., R.B. Amon, F.J. Storrs, and C.R. White, Jr. 1983. Phytophotodermatitis due to *Ruta graveolens*. Contact Dermatitis **9**(4):278-280.

207

REFERENCES

Hofmann, E., D. Schlee, and H. Reinbothe. 1969. On the occurrence and distribution of allantoin in Boraginaceae. Flora Abt. A Physiol. Biochem. **159(6)**:510-518.

Inya-agha, S.I., B.O. Oguntimein, E.A. Sofowora, and T.V. Benjamin. 1987. Phytochemical and antibacterial studies on the essential oil of *Eupatorium odoratum*. Int. J. Crude Drug Res. **25(1)**:49-52.

Islam, B.N. 1984. Pesticidal action of Neem and certain indigenous plants and weeds of Bangladesh. Schriftenr GTZ. **161**:263-290.

Jain, M.L. and S.R. Jain. 1972. Therapeutic utility of *Ocimum basilicum* var. *album*. Planta Med. **22**:66.

Janssen, A.M., N.L.J. Chin, J.J.C. Scheffer, and A. Baerheim Svendsen. 1986. Screening for antimicrobial activity of some essential oils by the agar overlay technique. Pharm. Weekbl. (Sci. Ed.) **8(6)**:289-292.

Jelliffe, D.B., G. Bras, and K.L. Stuart. 1954. The clinical picture of veno-occlusive disease of the liver in Jamaican children. Ann. Trop. Med. Parasitol **48**:386-396.

Jiménez Misas, C.A., N.M. Rojas Hernández, and A.M. López Abraham. 1979a. Contribution to the biological evaluation of Cuban plants. 5. Rev. Cub. Med. Trop. **31**:37-43.

_____. 1979b. Contribution to the biological evaluation of Cuban plants. 6. Rev. Cub. Med. Trop. **31**:45-51.

Jiravanit, P., S.U.T. Charoenkornvichit, U. Wongkrajang, P. Pungvicha, and P. Jaiard. 1985. Result of *Chromolaena odorata* (L.) K.&R. in accelerating the blood clotting process. Special topic: As a part of the requirement for the Bachelor degree in Pharmacy (1985), College of Pharmacy, Mahidol University, Bangkok, Thailand:31.

Kalyanasundaram, M. and C.J. Babu. 1982. Biologically active plant extracts as mosquito larvicides. Indian J. Med. Res. Suppl. **76**:102-106.

Kerr, K.M., T.J. Mabry, and S. Yoser. 1981. 6-hydroxy- and 6-methyoxyflavonoids from *Neurolaena lobata* and *N. macrocephala*. Phytochemistry **20**:791-794.

Khan, M.R., G. Ndaalio, M.H. Nkunya, H. Wevers, and A.N. Sawhney. 1980. Studies on African medicinal plants. Part 1. Preliminary screening of medicinal plants for antibacterial activity. Planta Med. Suppl. **40**:91-97.

Kholkute, S.D. and K.N. Udupa. 1976. Antiestrogenic activity of *Hibiscus rosa-sinensis* Linn. flowers. Indian J. Exp. Biol. **14(2)**:175-176.

_____, V. Mudgal, and P.J. Deshpande. 1976. Screening of indigenous medicinal plants for antifertility potentiality . Planta Med. **29**:151-155.

Kingsbury, J.M. 1964. *Poisonous plants of the United States and Canada*. Englewood Cliffs, New Jersey: Prentice-Hall, Inc. 507 pp.

REFERENCES

Kishore, N., N.K. Dubey, S.K. Singh, and S.N. Dixit. 1981. Fungitoxicity of some volatile natural products against human pathogenic fungi. Indian Perf. **25(3&4)**:1-3.

Kritsanapan, W. 1978. Phytochemical studies of *Cassia timoriensis [sic]* de Candolle and *C. grandis* L.. Master's thesis. Faculty of Pharmacy, Chulalongkorn University, Bangkok, Thailand, 1978. 105 pp.

Lavin, M. 1986. The occurrence of canavanine in seeds of the tribe Robinieae. Biochem. Syst. Ecol. **14(1)**:71-73.

Leatherdale, B.A., R.K. Panesar, G. Singh, T.W. Atkins, C.J. Bailey, and A.H.C. Bignell. 1981. Improvement in glucose tolerance due to *Momordica charantia* (Karela). Brit. Med. J. **282(6279)**:1823-1824.

Lima, O.G. de and I.L. D'Albuquerque. 1958. A simple method of extraction and purification of biflorine. Rev. Inst. Antibiot., Univ. Fed. Pernambuco Recife. **1**:7-9.

López Abraham, A.M., N.M. Rojas Hernández, and C.A. Jiménez Misas. 1981. Potential antineoplastic activity of Cuban plants. 4. Rev. Cubana Farm. **15(1)**:71-77.

López V., J.A. and Y.E. Hernández M. 1981. Isolation of cinnamic acid and sucrose in the fruit of *Cassia grandis* L. (Leguminosae). Ing. Cienc. Quim. **5(2)**:66.

Lorenzetti, B.B., G.E.P. Souza, S.J. Sarti, D.Santos Filho, and S.H. Ferreira. 1991. Myrcene mimics the peripheral analgesic activity of lemongrass tea. J. Ethnopharmacol. **34(1)**:43-48.

Louw, P.G.J. 1948. Lantadene A, the active principle of *Lantana camara*. 2. Isolation of lantadene B, and the oxygen functions of lantadene A and lantadene B. Onderstepoort J. Vet. Sci. Animal Ind. **23**:233-238.

Loveman, A.B. 1937. Leaf of *Aloe vera* in treatment of roentgen ray ulcers: Report on two additional cases. Arch. Dermatol. Syphilol. **36**:838.

Lowry, J.B. 1968. The distribution and potential taxonomic value of alkylated ellagic acids. Phytochemistry **7(10)**:1803-1813.

Lubieniecki, S. 1961. Photodermatosis due to contact with *Chenopodium*: Case report. Polski Tygodnik Lekarski **16(3)**:105.

Macfoy, C.A. and A.M. Sama. 1983. Medicinal plants in Pujehun district of Sierra Leone. J. Ethnopharmacol. **82**:215-223.

Malcolm, S.A. and E.A. Sofowora. 1969. Antimicrobial activity of selected Nigerian folk remedies and their constituent plants. Lloydia **32**:512-517.

Manchand, P.S. and J.F. Blount. 1978. Stereostructures of neurolenins A and B novel germacranolide sesquiterpenes from *Neurolaena lobata*. J. Org. Chem. **43**:4352.

Mancini, B. 1980. Pharmacognostic study of leaves and stems of *Wedelia paludosa* var. *vialis*, Compositae: Analysis of the essential oil. Rev. Cienc. Farm. **2**:61-76.

REFERENCES

Martinez, M.A. 1984. Medicinal plants used in a Totonac community of the Sierra Norte De Puebla: Tuzamapan De Galeana, Puebla, Mexico. J. Ethnopharmacol. **11(2)**:203-221.

Martinez-Crovetto, R. 1981. Fertility-regulating plants used in popular medicine in Northeastern Argentina. Parodiana **1(1)**:97-117.

Maruzzella, J.C., D. Scrandis, J.B. Scrandis, and G. Grabon. 1960. Action of odoriferous organic chemicals and essential oils on wood-destroying fungi. Plant Dis. Rept. **44**:789.

May, G. and G. Willuhn. 1978. Antiviral activity of aqueous extracts from medicinal plants in tissue cultures. Arzneim.-Forsch. **28(1)**:1-7.

McKenzie, R.A., F.P. Franke, and P.J. Dunster. 1987. The toxicity to cattle and bufadienolide content of six *Bryophyllum* species. Aust. Vet. J. **64(10)**:298.

Meuller-Oerlinghausen, F., W. Ngamwathana, and P. Kanchanapee. 1971. Investigation into Thai medicinal plants said to cure diabetes. J. Med. Ass. Thailand **54**:105-111.

Mishra, S.H. and S.C. Chaturvedi. 1978. Antibacterial and antifungal activity of alkaloid *[sic]* of *Sida rhombifolia*. Indian Drugs. **16**:61-63.

Morrison, E.Y.St.A.and M.E. West. 1985. The effect of *Bixa orellana* (Annatto) on blood sugar levels in the anaesthetized dog. West Indian Med. J. **34(1)**:38-42.

Moussu, R. 1925. Poisoning with grains of *Cassia occidentalis* L. is due to a toxic albumin. Compt. Rend. Soc. Biol. **92**:862-863.

Mowrey, D.B. and D.E. Clayson. 1982. Motion sickness, ginger and psychophisics. Lancet **20**:655-657.

Mukherjee, K.S. and P.K. Ghosh. 1978. Phytochemical studies on *Salvia coccinea* Linn.. J. Indian Chem. Soc. **55(3)**:292, 850.

Nagaty, H.F., M.A. Rifatt, and T.A. Morsy. 1959. Trials on the effect on dog *Ascaris* in vivo produced by the latex of *Ficus carica* and *Papaya carica* growing in Cairo gardens. Ann. Trop. Med. Parasitol. **53**:215.

Nahrstedt, A., U. Eilert, B. Wolters, and V. Wray. 1981. Rutacridone-epoxide, a new acridone alkaloid from *Ruta graveolens*. Z Naturforsch Ser. C. **36**:200-203.

Narayana L.L., I.T. Sundari, and M. Radhakrishnaiah. 1981. Chemotaxonomy of some Annonaceae. Curr. Sci. **50**:1079-1080.

Nascimento, S.C. do, J.F. de Méllo, and A. de A. Chiappeta. 1985. Cytotoxic agents: Experiments with KB cells. Rev. Inst. Antibiot., Univ. Fed. Pernambuco Recife **22(1/2)**:19-26.

_____, A. de A. Chiappeta, and R.M.O.C. Lima. 1990. Antimicrobial and cytotoxic activities in plants from Pernambuco, Brazil. Fitoterapia **61(4)**:353-355.

National Cancer Institute. 1976. Unpublished and confidential data. Nat. Cancer Inst. Central Files.

REFERENCES

Noble, I.G. 1947. Fruta bomba *(Carica papaya)* in hypertension. An. Acad. Cienc. Med. Fis. Nat. Habana. **85**:198.

Oguntimein, B.O. 1987. The terpenoids of *Annona reticulata*. Fitoterapia **58(6)**:411-413.

O'Hara, P.J. and K.R Pierce. 1974. Toxic cardiomyopathy caused by *Cassia occidentalis*. 2. Biochemical studies in poisoned rabbits. Vet. Pathol. **11(2)**:110-124.

Onawunmi, G.O. 1989. Evaluation of the antifungal activity of lemon grass oil. Int. J. Crude Drug Res. **27(2)**:121-126.

_____ and E.O. Ogunlana. 1986. A study of the antibacterial activity of the essential oil of lemon grass *(Cymbopogon citratus* (DC.) Stapf.). Int. J. Crude Drug Res. **24(2)**:64-68.

Pandey, D.K., H. Chandra, and N.N. Tripathi. 1982. Volatile fungitoxic activity of some higher plants with special reference to that of *Callistemon lanceolatus* DC.. Phytopathol. Z **105**:175-182.

Pandey, V.B., J.P. Singh, Y.V. Rao, and S.B. Acharya. 1982. Isolation and pharmacological action of heliotrine, the major alkaloid of *Heliotropium indicum* seeds. Planta Med. **45**:229-233.

Papavassiliou, M.J. and C. Eliakis. 1937. Rue as an abortifacient and poison. Ann. Med. Leg. **17**:993.

Paris, R.R. and H. Moyse. 1981. *Précis de Matière Médicale*. 2nd ed., rev. Vol. 2. Paris, France: Masson. 518 pp.

Pérez G., R.M., A. Ocegueda A., J.L. Muñoz L., J.G. Avila A., and W.W. Morrow. 1984. A study of the hypoglucemic *[sic]* effect of some Mexican plants. J. Ethnopharmacol. **12(3)**:253-262.

Pilcher, J.D. 1916. The action of various "female" remedies on the excised uterus of the guinea pig. J. Amer. Med. Ass. **67**:490.

Pongpan, A., W. Avirutnant, and P. Chumsri. 1983. Some Thai plants as substrates for microbial protein production. Madhidol Univ. J. Pharm. Sci. **10(1)**:15-18.

Pursglove, J.W. 1974. *Tropical Crops: Monocotyledons*. Volumes 1 and 2 combined. London: Longman Group Ltd. 607 pp.

Queiroz Neto, A. and I. Melito. 1990. Changes in sensitivity of the isolated guinea-pig vas deferens induced by a lyophilized *Phoradendron latifolium* leaf infusion. J. Ethnopharmacol. **28(2)**:183-189.

Raffauf, R.F., M.D. Menachery, P.W. Le Quesne, E.V. Arnold, and J. Clardy. 1981. Antitumor plants. 11. Diterpenoid and flavonoid constituents of *Bromelia pinguin* L.. J. Org. Chem. **46**:1094-1098.

Rai, M.K. and S. Upadhyay. 1988. Screening of medicinal plants of Chhindwara District against *Trichophyton mentagrophytes*: A causal organism of *Tinea pedis*. Hindustan Antibiot. Bull. **30(1/2)**:33-36.

Ray, P.G. and S.K. Majumdar. 1976. Antimicrobial activity of some Indian plants. Econ. Bot. **30**:317-320.

REFERENCES

Ribeiro, R. de A., F. de Barros, M.M.R. Fiuza de Melo, C. Muniz, S. Chieia, M. das Graças Wanderley, C. Gomes, and G. Trolin. 1988. Acute diuretic effects in conscious rats produced by some medicinal plants used in the state of Sao Paulo, Brazil. J. Ethnopharmacol. **24(1)**:19-29.

_____, M.M.R. Fiuza de Melo, F. de Barros, C. Gomes, and G. Trolin. 1986. Acute antihypertensive effect in conscious rats produced by some medicinal plants used in the state of Sao Paulo. J. Ethnopharmacol. **15(3)**:261-269.

Richter, E.R. and L.A. Vore. 1989. Antimicrobial activity of banana puree. Food Microbiol. **6(3)**:179-187.

Robineau, L., ed. 1991. *Hacia una farmacopea caribeña. Seminario TRAMIL 4 (Tela, Honduras, Noviembre 1989): Investigacion cientifica y uso popular de plantas medicinales en el caribe.* Santo Domingo, República Dominicana: enda-caribe. 387 pp.

Roig y Mesa, J.T. 1945. *Plantas medicinales, aromaticas o venenosas de Cuba.* Havana: Ministerio de Agricultura, Republica de Cuba. 872 pp.

Rojas Hernández, N.M., C.A. Jiménez Misas, A.M. López Abraham, and C. Hernández Suárez. 1981. Study of the inhibitory activity of plant extracts on microbial growth. Part 5. Rev. Cubana Farm. **15**:139-145.

Ross, S.A., N.E. El-Keltawi, and S.E. Megalla. 1980. Antimicrobial activity of some Egyptian aromatic plants. Fitoterapia **51**:201-205.

Saad, J.M., Y.H. Hui, J.K. Rupprecht, J.E. Anderson, J.F. Kozlowski, G.X. Zhao, K.V. Wood, and J.L. McLaughlin. 1991. Reticulatacin: A new bioactive acetogenin from *Annona reticulata* (Annonaceae). Tetrahedron **47(16/17)**:2751-2756.

Saksena, N. and H.H.S. Tripathi. 1985. Plant volatiles in relation to fungistasis. Fitoterapia **56(4)**:243-244.

Samuelsson, G., L. Borsub, A.L. Jayawardene, L. Falk, S. Ziemilis, and O. Nilsson. 1981. Screening of plants of the families *Loranthaceae* and *Viscaceae* for toxic proteins. Acta Pharm. Suecica **18**:179-184.

Savona, G., M. Bruno, M. Paternostro, J.L. Marco, and B. Rodriguez. 1982. Salviacoccin, a neo-clerodane diterpenoid from *Salvia coccinea*. Phytochemistry **21**:2563-2566.

Shah, A.H., S. Qureshi, M. Tariqu, and A.M. Ageel. 1989. Toxicity studies on six plants used in the traditional Arab system of medicine. Phytother. Res. **3(1)**:25-29.

Sharaf, A. 1969. Food plants as a possible factor in fertility control. Qual. Plant Mater Veg. **17**:153.

Siddhartha, P. and A.K.N. Chaudhuri. 1990. Anti-inflammatory action of *Bryophllyum pinnatum* leaf extract. Fitoterapia **61(6)**:527-533.

Sievers, A.F. W.A. Archer, R.H. Moore, and B.R. McGovern. 1949. Insecticidal tests of plants from tropical America. J. Econ. Entomol. **42**:549.

REFERENCES

Simon, O.R. and N. Singh. 1986. Demonstration of anticonvulsant properties of an aqueous extract of spirit weed (*Eryngium foetidum* L.). WI Med. J. **35**(2):121-125.

Simopoulos, A.P., H.A. Norman, J.E. Gillaspy, and J.A. Duke. 1992. Common purslane: A source of omega-3 fatty acids and antioxidants. J. Am. Coll. Nutr. **11**(4):374-382.

_____ and N. Salem, Jr. 1987. Purslane: A terrestrial source of omega-3 fatty acids. N. Engl. J. Med. **315**(13):833.

Singh, K.V. and R.K. Pathak. 1984. Effect of leaves [*sic*] extracts of some higher plants on spore germination of *Ustilago maydes* and *U. nuda*. Fitoterapia **55**(5):318-320.

Soytong, K., V. Rakvidhvasastra, and T. Sommartya. 1985. Effect of some medicinal plants on growth of fungi and potential in plant disease control. Abstr. 11th Conference of Science and Technology, Thailand Kasetsart University, Bangkok, Thailand, October 24-26, 1985. **1985**:361.

Spencer, C.F., F.R. Koniuszy, E.F. Rogers, J. Shavel Jr., N.R. Easton, E.A. Kaczka, F.A. Kuehl, Jr., R.F. Phillips, A. Walti, K. Folkers, C. Malanga, and A.O. Seeler. 1947. Survey of plants for antimalarial activity. Lloydia **10**:145-174.

Srivastava, Y.S. and P.C. Gupta. 1981. A new flavonol glycoside from seeds of *Cassia grandis*. Planta Med. **41**:400-402.

Standley, P.C. and J.A. Steyermark. 1946. Flora of Guatemala. Fieldiana: Botany. **24**(5):92, 265-266, 448-449.

_____. 1949. Flora of Guatemala. Fieldiana: Botany. **24**(6):111-112, 287-288, 399-400.

Sydiskia, R.J. and D.G Owen. 1987. *Aloe* emodin and other anthraquinones and anthraquinone-like compounds from plants virucidal against *Herpes simplex* viruses. Patent-U.S.-4, 670, 265. 7 pp.

Tezuka, H. and K. Kitabatake. 1980. Growth-inhibitory activity in *Papaya* latex against *Candida* species. Bull. Brew. Sci. **26**:47-49.

Tirimanna, A.S.L.. 1981. Annatto. 1. Preliminary data of the chemical composition. Colet. Inst. Technol. Aliment. 1980. **11**:89-96.

Tomas-Barberan, F.A., J.B. Harborne, and R. Self. 1987. Dimalonated anthocyanins from the flowers of *Salvia splendens* and *S. coccinea*. Phytochemistry **26**(10):2759-2760.

Tripathi, S.C. and S.N. Dixit. 1977. Fungitoxic properties of *Rosa chinensis*. Experientia **33**:207-209.

Upadhya, G.S., G. Narayanaswamy, and A.R.S. Kartha. 1974. Note on the comparative development of fatty acids in ripening seeds of 6 dicot species producing C16-C18 acid fats. Indian J. Agr. Sci. **44**:620.

213

REFERENCES

Van Den Berghe, D.A., M. Ieven, F. Mertens, A.J. Vlietinck, and E. Lammens. 1978. Screening of higher plants for biological activities. 2. Antiviral activity. J. Nat. Prod. **41**:463-467.

Venkataraman, S., T.R. Ramanujam, and V.S. Venkatasubbu. 1980. Antifungal activity of the alcoholic extract of coconut shell: *Cocos nucifera* Linn.. J. Ethnopharmacol. **2**(3):291-293.

Verhulst, H.L. and L.A. Page. 1962. *Lantana*. Bull. of Natl. Clearinghouse Pois. Contr. Cent. Feb.-Mar. **1962**:6.

Verpoorte, R. and P.P. Dihal. 1987. Medicinal plants of Surinam. 4. Antimicrobial activity of some medicinal plants. J. Ethnopharmacol. **21**:315-318.

Vieira, J.E.V., G.S.G. Barros, M.C. Medeiros, F.J.A. Matos, M.P. Souza, and M.J. Medeiros. 1968. Pharmacologic screening of plants from Northeast Brazil. 2. Rev. Brasil Farm. **49**:67-75.

Wanjari, D.G. 1983. Antihaemorrhagic activity of *Lantana camara*. Nagarjun. **27**(2):40-41.

Westbrooks, R.G. and J.W. Preacher. 1986. *Poisonous plants of Eastern North America.* Columbia, South Carolina: University of South Carolina Press. 226 pp.

Yamagishi, T., M. Haruna, X.Z. Yan, J.J. Chang, and K.H. Lee. 1989. Antitumor agents. 110. Bryophyllin B, a novel potent cytotoxic bufadienolide from *Bryophyllum pinnatum*. J. Nat. Prod. **52**(5):1071-1079.

Yang T.H. and M.Y. Cheng. 1987. The alkaloids of *Annona reticulata* L.. 2. Tai-Wan Yao Hsueh Tsa Chich **39**(3):195-201.

INDEX
OF SCIENTIFIC AND COMMON NAMES

INDEX

INDEX

INDEX

INDEX

ABOUT THE AUTHORS

Dr. Rosita Arvigo, D.N. has lived in Central America for 25 years and, throughout that time, has studied with various traditional healers. She is a practicing alternative physician, having received her degree from the Chicago National College of Naprapathy. She is President and a cofounder of the Ix Chel Tropical Research Foundation in Cayo, Belize, home of the Panti Mayan Medicine Trail, a "living museum" where many of Belize's useful plants can be observed in their natural setting.

Dr. Michael J. Balick, Ph.D. is a tropical botanist who received his doctorate from Harvard University. In the past two decades, he has carried out botanical and ethnobotanical studies in Central and South America, the Caribbean, Asia, and the Middle East. He is Director and Philecology Curator of Economic Botany at the Institute of Economic Botany of The New York Botanical Garden. He serves as Chairman and is a cofounder of the Ix Chel Tropical Research Foundation.

ABOUT THE ILLUSTRATOR

Laura Evans is an artist, illustrator, and gardener in Sandy Hook, Connecticut. She received her Bachelor of Fine Arts degree in 1980 from Northern Kentucky University and has exhibited in galleries in Kentucky, Ohio, and Connecticut. She would like to thank her husband, Robert Pawlikowski, whose photographs were used to help illustrate many of the plants in this book.